The Mouth Trap:
the butt stops here!
Low-Carb Edition

A happy, healthy way to eat!

by Pam Young

ISBN 978-0-9833880-4-3

9 780983 388043

Don't miss my other great books:

The Sidetracked Sisters' Happiness File
by Pam Young and Peggy Jones

Sidetracked Home Executives: From Pigpen to Paradise
by Pam Young and Peggy Jones

The Sidetracked Sisters Catch Up on the Kitchen
by Pam Young and Peggy Jones

I'm Okay...but You Have a Lot of Work to Do!
by Pam Young and Peggy Jones

Get Your Act Together: A 7-Day Get-Organized Program For The Overworked, Overbooked, and Overwhelmed
by Pam Young and Peggy Jones

The GOOD Book: Get Out Of Debt*
by Pam Young

The Mouth Trap: the butt stops here!*
by Pam Young

* only be available as an audio/eBook

Dedication

This book is dedicated to the word "mmmm." Okay, I know it's not really a word, but we all use it from time to time especially when we've tasted something yummy or smelled good food cooking like a turkey roasting, or cinnamon rolls baking. "Mmmm."

I think we should use the word as much as we can because it's a natural sound that when we make it, it enhances our experience, whatever it is. I had a very wise meditation teacher help me find my natural "ohm" sound when I was in my early twenties. He said, "Tell me what delights you." The first thought out of my mind was, "Puppies." So he said, "When you pick up a puppy and snuggle it, do you say anything?" I thought for a second and answered, "Yeah, I say 'ohhhhhh.' "That's YOUR ohm sound and if you'll use it in meditation when you breathe out you will become centered very quickly." How wise! We really do have a personal ohm sound and a personal mmm and the more we use both of them the happier and more content we can be.

From now on when you hear yourself say, "mmm," really enjoy the sensation. Let your "mmm" enhance the taste. It happens to me frequently when I'm in a nice restaurant and taste a new spice or flavor I don't usually cook with at home. Whenever I take a bite that deserves an "mmm," I savor it by closing my eyes and really getting into the experience. One bite can elicit several "mmms," and that's okay. If you get hit with an "mmm" in a restaurant you'll need to use discretion. You don't want to make a scene like Meg Ryan did in the movie *When Harry Met Sally*, but I trust you'll use good judgment.

I'd also like to dedicate this book to all of you who have struggled with a weight problem. I know your tears of frustration. I've heard your cries of "It's not fair," "Why me?" and "What's wrong with me?" I've felt the self-hate, the embarrassment and the sense of failure. I've been disappointed and angry with myself and I've given up so many times I can't count them. I love each and every one of you and our struggles have inspired me to find a new way! Struggle is such an ugly word and it *never* works. Today you can decide to stop struggling and try a new approach. This new approach is unlike any you've ever thought of, because in your past you connected weight loss with torture distress, misery and suffering and of course failure.

This approach is infused with joy and appreciation for life. This new approach can be like going on a dream vacation you've always looked forward to. As I embarked on this new way to eat and live, I took with me all the women in my life that I know personally who have *struggled* with a weight problem (and there are many) and I imagined them with me in spirit at every turn. I adore every one of them, from my grandmother to Oprah and all those in between. I couldn't wait to be able to share my joyous findings with these women and those of you whom I don't know.

I'm bursting with secrets and it's FINALLY time to share them with you. Even though I can't personally hear you, I'll be delighted with every "mmm" you utter as you join me in this exciting adventure. I'll be celebrating every pound you lose, every plateau you reach and every loving moment you spend being kind and easy with yourself.

Table of Contents

Introduction

It took me two years to write *The Mouth Trap: the butt stops here!* because it was a diary of my weight loss which took two years. After I lost 35 pounds and polished my writing, I released the book in January of 2011.

I have learned so much since then that I was compelled to rewrite much of it. If you read the first edition you know that I said, "This is not a diet book. It doesn't tell you what to eat, it tells you how to mind whatever diet you're on." This new book will still help you mind, but it will now tell you what to eat.

The old book also advocated Weight Watchers because at the time I truly believed it was a nutritious plan to follow. I don't anymore. Now, let's get to the NEW book.

My mouth gets me into more trouble than any other hole in my body. Sometimes it's because of what comes out of it, but mostly it's been because of what goes in. That's why the title to my book is The Mouth Trap: *the butt stops here!*

Unless you're hooked up to an intravenous feeding contraption that continues to pump too much food into your system, the size of your body is entirely due to your mouth's ability to open and let the food that has made you weigh more than you like, to come in and "accumulate."

You could rationalize that your size is due to genetics, but in the end, your ancestors are hardly to blame for your mouth opening. You can argue that your condition is due to your age and whine that the older you get, the harder it is to lose, but it's no harder to open and close your mouth now than it was when you were eighteen or thirty. You can blame your problem on stress, or not enough money or too little time or the fast food industry, or, or, or... The bottom line is... you are either in control of your mouth or you aren't. You are the one who opens it and if you've opened it to the wrong kinds of food (mainly sugars, starches and grains, yes grains), right now you have a fabulous opportunity to use this problem as a window to get to know the "opener" in a stunning way you never dreamt of before.

I wrestled with whether I was qualified to write this book. I can't make any claims such as, "I lost 200 pounds on this weight-loss plan." All I can say is that I lost 35 pounds in two years, gained ten back in six months, lost the ten in one year and have finally remained at my goal weight ever since, using the psychological tools I created and knowledge about the science behind what we've been *told* is a healthy diet and what really is one.

We've been so brain-washed in our society to go for fast results that you are probably thinking, '35 pounds lost over three and a half years, what's the big deal?' It IS a big deal. I found out that losing weight slowly gives a person inner growing room. When you take the pressure off by eliminating a deadline, you'll find the journey is much easier, more fun and the results will serve you the rest of your life. With my tools you will enjoy and appreciate each plateau you reach.

Instead of embarking on a diet with the same urgency as induced labor, you are going to take it easy this time and lose naturally, with the primary goal of getting to know more about you. The secondary goal is to lose no more than a pound a week and keep it off for life. You'll find out why I didn't keep the 35 pounds off and what happened after this book was finished (the first time). Something unexpected came into my life and changed it drastically forever.

This book is for people whose lifestyles and circumstances have resulted in unwanted pounds over time and who have dieted in the past only to gain it all back and then some more. It's also for those who have lost weight, because they have dieted and now want to maintain that desired weight.

My husband and I were cheerleading partners at Fort Vancouver High. In the forty-five years since he'd lifted me up on his shoulders, I'd put on forty-five pounds. Hey that's only one pound a year! That's not even two ounces a month! Oh, and the earrings I wore in high school? Still fit. Though I don't weigh 120, I love what I weigh now for my age. And I can't wait to share what I have learned.

Here are a few hints of what's to come:

You'll be guided through the grieving process of losing your dear friend (that love of carbohydrates). I'm not going to tell you that you can never have cake or potatoes ever again, but I can say you won't want them ever again. Honest! I'll show you how to get through all the traditional holidays that emphasize the use of sugar.

You'll learn how I got hold of the ultimate motivation to finally lose weight and how this epiphany totally changed my way of thinking, which gave me the motivation to succeed.

You'll learn how to take advantage of an impending event like a class reunion or wedding to increase your weight loss.

You'll learn how to bounce out of denial forever. (If you don't think you're in denial, step on the scales.) What I learned will be one of your most effective tools. It's easier than you think.

You'll learn to gradually build a new vocabulary concerning food.

You'll discover you only need to be accountable to yourself.

You'll learn about the most powerful instrument I discovered. I'll show you in detail how to make that instrument work for you.

You'll learn to see through the eyes of a child and turn losing weight into the most fun and meaningful projects of your life and you'll gain a new best friend along the way.

You'll love what the supreme experts (children) have to say about your best source of joy. You'll delight in their suggestions for having fun.

I'll give you the secret I discovered for instantly eliminating craving for sugar and starches (and it turned out to be scientific).

You'll learn the five simple steps for guiding yourself out of stress. Reduce stress! Reduce eating! Reduce weight!

You'll learn how I made what I call a "Wake-up Collar" to remind me why I was on this journey in the first place. You will be shocked at its impact!

Your eyes will be opened to inventive ways to use your imagination to personalize your weight loss adventure.

You'll be given one thought that can cause you to lose up to ten pounds in this next year. Just one little thought.

You'll learn a new definition of a Consumer Report and how powerful it can be in helping you lose weight.

You'll learn why you'll never count calories again and how the freedom that comes from that will raise your happiness quotient.

I'll share with you why I should now weigh 288 pounds, but have maintained my goal weight for more than a year.

You won't believe how simple it is and how it will help you to stay on track when you get that "It's not fair" feeling.

You'll study strategies from those who have lost a lot of weight and kept if off for years. They have "been there and done that" and will serve as an inspiration to you.

You'll find out how judging others is a sure way to stay overweight. Here is a hint. Don't look twice.

The most important discovery is that your weight problem is a blessing and a window to get as healthy as you can and to know and love who you are.

If you know me, you know my slogan: "Make it fun and it will get done." This entire book is filled with fun ideas to help you achieve your weight-loss goals. It's meant to turn things you formerly dreaded into enjoyable and pleasant adventures.

Meet My Co-Author

Now, I'd like to introduce you to my co-author, Nelly. She will share her thoughts with you throughout this book. Nelly, would you like to say something to the ladies?

"Hello."

"Can you tell everyone just a little bit about yourself?"

"I'm Nelly and I'm nine years old. I love to play and I love to eat in restaurants where people serve you and when they put your plate down they say, 'Enjoy.'

I used to love baked potatoes with sour cream and butter and chocolate covered doughnuts and Burger King Whoppers and pizza and ice cream and fresh warm bread wi. . ."

"Nelly?"

"Huh?"

"You know this is a book to help people cut down on carbohydrates and lose weight?"

"Yeah?"

"Well, maybe you shouldn't be running through all those foods that were so tempting to you in the past."

"Well, just because I don't want that stuff anymore doesn't mean I can't talk about it. It's kinda fun."

"Point taken. And what's the big lesson we're going to teach in this book, anyway?"

"That when we eat what we ate for a bajillion years we're never hungry, so we're happy."

"That's right."

You'll learn more about who Nelly is in the first chapter: *Have Fun Losing Weight with Your Own Best Friend*. More importantly, you'll learn how to meet, love and partner up with the Nelly in your life, for the rest of your life.

This is not a diet book. There are a million diet books on the market and, unfortunately for most people, those diets don't work because we usually go on them to lose weight.

If you follow what Nelly and I reveal in this book, you will be adopting a lifestyle. It doesn't matter how much weight you have to lose or how old you are. Someone who is 65 with 25 pounds to lose can change her mind as easily as a 25 year-old with 65 pounds to lose. Changing your mind is what this book is really all about.

It's filled with "AHA!" moments and you'll discover you can be successful with achieving your goal weight and staying at it for the rest of your life. You'll be pleasantly surprised how fun it is to lose weight this time, your last time!

You'll love the drama Nelly adds, and you'll be amazed at how powerful your imagination is and the effect it can have on your weight loss program.

Whether you have 20 pounds or 200 pounds to lose, whether it's the first 20 or the last 20, this book will change your life. Your old way of dieting will be gone and your excess baggage will go with it.
The huge difference is this time you are going to be aware of a new friend (who has been your worst enemy). That friend will be involved with every bite you'll take for the rest of your life: YOU; YOU, the opener.

For now, just know you are on your way to a lighter life.

Enjoy!

Chapter One:
Have Fun Losing Weight
with Your Own Best Friend

You briefly met Nelly in the Introduction and you're probably wondering where she came from and who she is. She is my *inner* child. I got acquainted with her in 2002 and I've grown to have a daily relationship with her.

That partnership is why I was able to get out of debt and write about it in *The GOOD Book*, (good stands for *Get Out Of Debt*). And it's primarily because of our connection that I successfully lost the weight.

All of your self-improvement plans, whether they be weight loss, organization, getting out of debt or a number of other issues are influenced by and are dependent on your relationship with the most important person in your life. . .YOU.

Whether you are aware of the inner child aspect of yourself or not, you have one who has been with you since you left your childhood years. Your inner child will also be with you as long as you live because you were created to have her in your life forever.

In *The GOOD Book* I had some dialogue that has really helped people grasp the concept of having an inner child. I decided I should share it with you here. I want you to pretend you're a guy about 40 years old and you hear the phone ring.

"Ring, ring, ring?"

"Carl, here, what's up?"

"Hi Carl, guess who?"

"Uhhh, I don't know, say somethin' else."

"Well, does Aspen ring a bell?"

"Aspen? Who is this?"

"It's Michelle."

"Michelle? Michelle Aspen?"

"No, silly, Michelle Rockford, Aspen **Square**."

"Michelle Rockford, Aspen Square? Oh yeah! Hey you're a great skier!"

"Yeah, we did a little more than ski together."

"Yeah, we did! What can I do ya for?"

Clears throat, "Well, it was nine years ago today that we were, you know, together?"

"Wow, it doesn't seem that long ago!"

"I know, but guess what?"

"What?"

"You've got a kid and I can't take care of it anymore."

"A kid?"

"Yeah, I'm done! It's your turn now. Oh, and one thing you should know. The kid is overweight and you're gonna need to figure out what to do or it's gonna like end up in the circus if you know what I mean."

If you haven't had a relationship with your inner child, to suddenly find out you have one can be a shock, like poor Carl had. I hope the conversation between Carl and Michelle helps you to see the position you're in right now.

See, your *inner child* as having the weight problem and think how you would handle a "real" overweight child if you were put in its care. We, as women, are nurturers. Have you ever noticed how many women in nurturing positions are overweight?

I think it's because they give all their focus and caring to others, neglecting their own well-being. If you're a nurturing, caring person and you are overweight, all you have to do is set an intention to focus on your inner child.

Would you give that child unhealthy foods? Would you let it eat sugar on a daily basis? Would you let it get de-hydrated? Drink alcohol? Eat at ten o'clock at night?

When you become a kind, loving and nurturing parent to your inner child, the weight problem will disappear. That's why I said, the first goal in this book is to get you to use this problem as an opportunity to get to know, love and take care of YOU. Your little one is waiting for you.

You already know there is more to you than meets the "I."

If the concept of an inner child isn't easy for you to get your head around, think about this: Who is the "I" and who is "myself" in the following statements?

I felt sorry for myself
I was beside myself
I asked myself
I beat myself up
I promised myself
I'm too hard on myself
I amazed myself

I let myself go (if you let yourself go, you can get yourself back)
I need to take time to find myself
I fought with myself

I learned about Nelly at a very low time in my life. I was buried in almost $27,000.00 of credit card debt and was given the opportunity to write a humorous, "how to" book about financial organization. That book would put me back in the black, but it would've been the phoniest book ever written! I'd have to say to my readers, "Here's how to organize your finances and get out of debt, write a clever book about how to do that." What a ridiculous notion and I knew I wouldn't be able to do that.

One night, in the middle of a financial nightmare I woke up with a start! It was 2:00 am. I went into my home office and sat at my computer and cried. I started to pray and I asked God, "What is wrong with me?" I'd read a bunch of books on financial organization, how to get out of debt and how to budget, and I knew I'd have to fix things, but I didn't want to do it. After a bit of silence the answer came in the form of a question: "How old have you been acting when it comes to your finances?" I wasn't prepared to be questioned! This Questioner had some nerve! I was shocked, but it made me think.

My financial behavior was that of about a nine year old. That's when I realized if I were going to write a helpful book about being financially solvent, I'd have to fix my financial situation by addressing this immature part of me. My Questioner told me to get to know this part of me, name her and write the book from that part of me to that part of those who were in a similar situation. How brilliant is that?

I named her Nelly after Nelly Olson on the television show, *Little House on the Prairie*, because, when I first met her, she was a brat. Slowly over time she has become such a good little girl and today she is hardly ever a brat. If your inner child is a brat, don't despair! With some tender, loving care she will blossom into an angel.

Over the last eight years, I have been corresponding with thousands of women through my website and I've learned so much. For one thing, I originally named my website The Brat Factor because, as I said, I was dealing with a downright brat! The term offended thousands of women and gradually as I came to love and respect this adorable part of me, I now agree that calling your inner child a brat does not serve you well.

As a Christian, I was a bit concerned about whether or not this work with an inner child was scriptural. Then I remembered what St. Paul said in Romans, Chapter 7, verse 15: For I do not know what I do; and I do not do the thing which I want, but I do the thing which I hate. That is exactly what I do.

Then he goes on to say in verses 17, 18, 19 and 20:
17: Now then it is not I who do it, but sin which dominates me.

18: Yet I know that it does not fully dominate me (that is in my flesh); but as far as good is concerned, the *choice* is easy for me to make, but to *do* it is difficult for me.

19: For it is not the good that I wish to do, that I do; but it is the evil that I do not wish to do, that I do.

20: Now if I do that which I do not wish, then it is not I who do it, but the sin which dominates me.

It's so nice to know I'm in good company. I love that Paul said it's easy to decide to do something, but then when it's time to do what we decide, unless we can fully dominate that little inner child who needs guidance, it is difficult to change so we can do the good we want to do.

I'm going to make a claim that contradicts the latest pop psychology tenant touting accountability: You DON'T have to be accountable to anyone but yourself.

Accountability can come from having a daily relationship with your inner child. I created a document I call the Weekly Progress Report and while I was losing weight, I wrote down Nelly's thoughts regarding food throughout the day every day. Thoughts like, 'Do you want some cheese or wine?' (When that thought came to me in the first couple of weeks, it struck me funny! One of the rules I'd made was no wine or cheese. The fact that Nelly gave me a choice of two forbidden items was typical of her sneaky ways.)

When I wrote that thought down on the Weekly Progress Report, Nelly felt as though she'd been written up. She hated seeing her thought in print! I had discovered a powerful tool to keep her in check. (I think it goes back to seeing teachers write the names of misbehaving children up on the blackboard). This self-accountability document proved to be one of the single most important tools I used along the way. You'll find the Weekly Progress Report in the Appendix.

Any suggestions I make please take them as just that. Do whatever works for you. I suggest weighing yourself at a consistent hour of the morning if you choose to weigh yourself every day. I suggest recording your weight once a week. At the beginning of each new week, write your weight on the Weekly Progress Report. You'll find instructions on how to use the report in Chapter Five: *Your Very Own Rules.*

Getting to know and love your inner child is paramount in my program. To get started, here's all you have to do: First, pick a name you love for her. (Be sure it's an endearing name, one that makes you smile.) I wish now

I'd named Nelly a name that didn't conjure up a brat, but, oh well, it doesn't mean "brat" to me now.

Second, as you read the next paragraph read as if you are saying this to your inner child. After you hear it (it ends with a question), pause the recording and listen for a response from yourself. You will get one in the form of a thought. That thought is coming straight from your inner child!

"Hi little one, I know you're there and I love you. I'm so sorry I've ignored you for such a long time, but I got busy with this thing called being a grown-up. Remember when I was your age and we played 'grown-up?' It was so much fun! What happened? You probably don't know because it's your job to stay young. Here's what I think happened. I wasn't ready to take on the responsibilities of being all grown up. I grew up too fast and put you aside. I've ignored you, until now. So let's get to know each other and let's agree to lose this weight together. So what do you think?"

If you draw a blank, start a dialogue like I just did and then think of another question. Perhaps ask something you've been wondering about lately. Once you receive an answer, tell your inner child you are sorry you've ignored her, ask her forgiveness, thank her and tell her you love her.

The rest of this book is written to both you and your inner child. You are no longer alone. You really never were. You just didn't know this part of YOU was so important. I'd like you to go to the store and buy a pretty card that says *I Love You* on the front or you can make your own. You can frame it if you'd like, and I want you to put it at your kitchen sink. (Your family will think you put it there because you love them and that's fine. However, you'll know the real meaning of the sign. It's from you to you.) The most vital notion to remember is to make this

14

relationship fun and loving. You'll see what happened to Nelly and me during this entire journey. As I said in the introduction she is the one who made this fun. She is very creative and she sees through the eyes of a child. That's where your new eyes are going to come from.

The very first order of business is to have a meeting with your inner child. You'll need time alone for this. Set the timer for 15 minutes and ask her what she loves, who she loves and what she'd like to do for fun (besides eat). The list can be on-going and as she comes up with more thoughts in the future, write them down in a note book just for all your favorite things. Nelly would you tell about our session?

"Pam sat down with me and had me tell her what I love, who I love, where I like to go and what I like to do. She turned the things I love into "rewards" (because I don't get to do them if I don't mind). Here are some of my rewards (off the top of my head): playing computer games, reading a good novel, playing with the neighbor's puppy, playing with Pam's grandchildren, singing with a chorus, playing in my garden, calling Marci, Joni, Carole, Shelly or LouAnn just to laugh and talk, writing on my "secret" novel, taking a bubble bath, getting a pedicure, manicure, going to meditation class, sculpting, taking a nap."

Your little one will come up with her own list and it may not have any of the items that are on Nelly's. Here is a note and a rather extensive list of things to do from one of my on-line friend's inner child.

> *Dear Pam and Nelly,*
> *My mom and I are just now starting to talk.*
> *When you first suggested that we meet, my*
> *mom thought she was supposed to meet me and*
> *help me to grow up. I didn't like that one bit!*
> *But now Mom understands that me being a kid*

is good for both of us, so I am ready to start talking to her again.

Mom and I were never allowed to be a kid, so I am bored a lot, but neither Mom nor I know what to do for fun. So, today Mom suggested that we call in our expert teachers, her real kids. Mom had them make lists of fun stuff that they like to do to give us some ideas.

The lists were great and they really helped get me started thinking of some really fun things for me and Mom to do (I think we will probably invite the outer kids to do some of the fun stuff with us).

-go to the fair
-watch TV
-cook
-ride an airplane
-ride on a ship
-visit Florida
-go to the beach
-grow a garden
-go see The Nutcracker Ballet
-go see Swan Lake
-go to the Library
-play Tetris
-go to Hobby Lobby
-tour the fire station
-go to the book store
-go skating
-go ice skating
-write stories
-play with dolls
-play dress up
-play with new hair styles
-color my hair (I want big chunky crayon purple highlights, mom is a little nervous about that. . .hopefully we can find a fun compromise. I

talked her into cutting her hair really short last year and she liked it.)
-get new hair accessories to try
-take a trip to Ireland
-go on a honeymoon with my dh
-buy lingerie and actually wear it
-visit the rain forest
-decorate for the holidays. . .especially Christmas and Halloween
-set off fireworks
-play video games
-play pirates with pretend swords
-play with trucks
-wear twirly skirts
-wear pretty jewelry
-be in a play
-play with clay / Play Doh
-paint
-draw
-do Caligraphy
-ride bikes
-go to Play World
-paint my nails
-go to the Zoo
-go to the museum
-go to the Science Museum
-go to the playground / park
-go visit Grandma
-go for a walk
-go on a scavenger hunt
-play in the rain
-play in the fountain
-take bubble baths
-swim
-take dance classes
-play board games
-visit friends
-gymnastics
-curl up and read a good book
-play outside

-hunt Easter Eggs
-rake leaves and jump in them
-surprise and be surprised
-play with siblings
-run through the sprinkler
-backyard water slide
-treasure hunt
-build with Legos
-buy toys at the store
-play Yahtzee
-play Monopoly
-find pretty leaves
-go on nature walks
-bird watching
-watch the sunset/sunrise
-cook outside
rearrange the furniture
-redecorate
-have pretty flowers on the table and over the sink
-snuggle with my sweetie
-read good books with the kids (not stuffy old books that mom thinks we SHOULD read for school, but fun books)
-play music
-sing

BTW, I haven't told my mom what my name is, so I can't tell you, it would ruin the surprise.

I especially enjoy getting emails from an inner child; it always shows the light-heartedness we tend to lose when we grow up.

Also in this session start a list of your favorite sights, sounds, smells, tastes and tactile sensations and even a list of your favorite thoughts. Remember in the *Sound of Music* when Maria sang *My Favorite Things*? The kids were afraid of the storm and she got them to forget about it. Also, think of an event in your life that was spectacular. What came to my mind for me was the birth of my first child. I can still feel the love that engulfed me and changed my life forever. If I take the time I can see that helpless infant, hold him in my mind's eye, smell him, hear his crying and remember how content he was nursing for the first time. Start a note book of Your Favorite Things. (I call mine my Happiness First Aid Kit.) Write down your memories and as more come to you add them. This session is extremely important because you are creating an arsenal of weapons to use against the negative thoughts that will undoubtedly come up on your journey to a lighter life.

About Thoughts

If you want to change a negative circumstance, you have to change the negative behavior that caused the circumstance. In order to change the behavior that caused the circumstance, you have to change the *thinking* behind the behavior. We think approximately 60,000 thoughts a day. That means much of our thinking is subconscious, under-the-radar of our conscious mind. We are wired to create habitual thought patterns so we can experience right now to the fullest. What a blessed gift that we were created to be able to establish habits. However, there's a dark side to that gift.

We can so easily slip into habitual behavior that can ruin our quality of life. No one consciously chooses to live in a dump, become a drug addict, ruin a marriage, go deeply into debt or become obese. Again they are under-the-radar choices. If you have established good habits, the adult part of you has been in charge. If you have a multitude of bad habits, your inner child has been running the show while you ignored her.

It's the negative thought *patterns* we want to change. Imagine those thought patterns to be like a parade of thoughts. There's a Grand Marshal just like in a real parade and that Grand Marshal thought is the "theme" thought that gathers and leads all the similar patterned thoughts it needs to get you to start marching right toward the freezer for a bowl of ice cream when you've decided you're going to lose 50 pounds this year. If you let the parade run its course, you could "wake up" to watching *Dancing with the Stars*, with an empty bowl on your stomach. Then you'd beat yourself up, put yourself down and start all over again by letting the next parade march right under your nose.

Your job, then, is to become aware of the parade before you join it. You have the power to ambush the parade that leads to self-indulgent and self-defeating behavior, by stopping the Grand Marshal (it's really your inner child) while the parade is in the "organizing" stage. (You can't behave without thinking even though it's under-the-radar thinking.) When you learn to recognize the "voice" of your inner child, you will be in a position of authority. Sort of like how the mayor of a city would confront a parade organizer who didn't have a permit.

"Excuse me, do you have a permit for this parade?"

"Uh, I didn't know I needed one."

"Yes, we don't allow parades without permits. You all need to go home."

You'll be amazed at the power you have to disperse the parade of thoughts! All it takes is a different thought or change of activities. This is the time to call in your arsenal of good thoughts. Most of the time I recognize Nelly's voice and depending on how determined she is, I have been able to change her mind with just a little distraction to divert her attention.

During my journey, Jacob one of my grandsons, had open-heart surgery. After being at the hospital all day with the family I came home and wanted a glass of wine. Wine was not on my food list, so I knew this was Nelly. Here's what

I did. I poured a tall glass of water and put ice in it (I know she loves that) and I sat in my chair in the living room where we read and I said,

"What's up baby girl?"

"Jacob."

"I know it was hard to see him in pain with tubes hooked to him."

"Peggy."

"I know we're worried about her taking care of herself. She's such a good mama and this is very hard for her and it's hard for us because I'm her mama. But everything is going to be just fine. All is well. We just need to let go and put it in God's hands. Now let's just sit here and sip our water and look out at the birds eating their seeds and watch the wind blowing in the trees. All is well. I love you."

As I sat in the chair for about ten minutes and drank my water and began to breathe nice, big even breaths, I realized it was water and oxygen I needed, not wine. To allow yourself ten minutes to breath and drink water is so much better than a glass of wine could ever be. Whenever we look for comfort outside ourselves we will never find it. It's not in food, it's not in wine it's not at the mall, it's within.

I will repeat this many times in this book: Discipline is remembering what you REALLY want. When you decide to change something in your life, the most important thing you must do is to have good reasons. In Chapter Five: *Your Very Own Rules*, I go into great detail on this subject. As you'll learn, if you and your inner child don't agree on what you really want and WHY you want it, this journey to lose weight and get healthy will come to a dead end. If you're not in agreement, as time passes your inner child will use every trick in her bag to cause you to succumb to self-defeating behavior which would ultimately sabotage your good intentions. What do you REALLY want? You want to live in a happy, healthy body that's easy to play in and looks good too.

When your inner child gets fussy with you these are the steps I recommend.

1. Stop what you are doing and listen.
2. Acknowledge her thought. If she wants something high in carbohydrates, acknowledge that she wants it.
3. As you plan your response get a glass of water and set the timer for two minutes (if that is possible).
4. Melt a tablespoon of butter and pour it over some cooked broccoli or cauliflower.
5. Sit, breathe deeply and remind her while drinking the water and eating the vegetable smothered in butter, what the reason is you are on this diet. You are not a subsidiary of U-Haul.
6. End the encounter by thanking her for minding, praise her for something she's done that's good, and tell her you love her.

As time goes on you'll be able to talk with her without stopping what you are doing, but in the beginning it helps to give her your full undivided attention. In the weeks to come you will have successes and failures but through it all if you will promise to maintain an open and honest relationship with your inner child you will win. I found that in the weeks I didn't lose weight those were weeks when Nelly needed more attention and didn't get it from me.

In my final diet, one of the most important lessons that came out of the experience at my tender age of 68 was what I call the 'plateau talk.' I had to have it many times with Nelly. It's similar to a real child asking, "Are we there yet?" on a long road trip. Whenever you've been discouraged with your weight loss results while on a diet, you can be sure it was the voice of your inner child that was fussing. Children are impatient and they don't like to have to wait for things to happen and your inner child is no exception. (I purposely planned to lose the weight gradually. I took 42 weeks to lose 25 pounds and another year to lose the last ten.) The plateau talks went something like this:

Nelly, "I did so good this week, I didn't argue and I DIDN'T LOSE A POUND!!!! WHAHHH!!!"

"I know but just think we didn't gain and we aren't trying to lose by a certain date. We're not on some big loser television show, so just enjoy what we've lost so far. It's just fine."

"BUT I'M MAD! I wanted to lose a pound and I didn't and I did so good. It's not fair! I DON'T WANT TO DO THIS ANYMORE. I'M QUITTING! WHAHHH!!"

Impatience is one of the biggest lessons we need to learn in life. When it comes to changing something as significant as your body and your health, I really believe that impatience is one of the greatest causes of failure to reach your goal. You didn't gain the weight overnight and you're not going to lose it overnight. If you think about all the diets you've been on, for each one you started you had to have quit one. Be easy and kind with yourself. When you catch yourself being impatient this is a golden opportunity to work with yourself to relax and look at the positive. Just think, as good parents we know in order to help our children through their difficulties we have to listen to what they're saying and help them understand that everything will be alright. You have to be your own cheerleader.

The other significant reason for failure with a diet, over time is what you've been eating. It was because of this factor that I was compelled to re-write this book. The impatience you've displayed in the past has a great deal to do with something that isn't your fault! You've been told by those in high places to eat an unhealthy diet; one that has been starving you and at the same time has made you fat! The combination of a healthy relationship with your inner child and a healthy diet is going to rock your world!

Assignment for Chapter One:

Meet and name your inner child.

Get a notebook and start your Happiness First Aid Kit notebook.

Buy a card or make a sign that says, I love you and post it at your kitchen sink.

Chapter Two:
A Big Fat Lie

On May 1, 2011 an unexpected package came from Amazon Books.

"Hmmm, I didn't order a book?"

When I opened it, I really knew I hadn't ordered it! The title was, *"Why We Get Fat and What To Do About it,"* by Gary Taubes, an award-winning science writer for the New York Times. Why would I buy a book with that title? I wasn't fat anymore! My first thought when I saw the bright red cover was, 'Thank God, for once I don't need to lose weight.' That thought came from the fact that I had spent the previous two years losing weight so I could launch my book *The Mouth Trap: the butt stops here!* By May, 1, 2011 it had been out for 5 months. I had made a promise to myself and my readers that until I lost 35 pounds going by my own advice in that book, it would not be released. I gradually lost the weight over a two-year period, (I thought it would take a year) and on January 17, 2010 I stepped on the scale and it said, "It's a go!" We released the book the next day.

What happened in the next four months will be a confession.

Once the excitement of the book launch set in and sales were doing very well, Nelly began to fuss. By following the calories-in/calories-out theory whereby 3,500 calories equals a pound, my guess is I ate an extra 7000 calories a month after the book release. That's approximately 233 calories every day more than I should have eaten to maintain my weight. By the end of April, 2011, I'd gained 10 pounds and Nelly was feeling trapped and nasty!

"Why'd you go and write that dumb book anyway? Now we HAVE to diet the whole rest of our life and I'll NEVER, NEVER, NEVER get a cinnamon roll or cake and ice cream or candy canes at Christmas, or …."

"Nelly, calm down, you know we can lose this ten pounds, we just have to start paying more attention and using all the wonderful tools you and I developed! You know they work and we really had fun, remember?"

"No I don't want to play prison anymore, or pretend I'm at a Fat Camp and Oprah's there to play with and I don't want to keep track of all the calories I turn down. I want ice cream now."

Following Weight Watcher's advice I burned approximately 500 calories six days a week walking religiously around the high hills in my neighborhood and I kept my calorie intake to 1800 a day. If I'd get sick and didn't walk, every seven days I was off the streets, I gained a pound, unless I cut back my calorie intake to 1200 calories.

I couldn't blame Nelly. I felt trapped by my own advice and by relaxing just a few rules here and there, skipping my walk once in a while, I was gradually gaining again and I did NOT want to be a hypocrite. There's nothing enlightening about touting a weight-loss book when you're over-weight. I was in serious trouble and that feeling of being a hypocrite was hanging on my back like a python squeezing every ounce of joy out of me. I felt stuck, but determined to read my own advice again and re-remember what kept me inspired through the two years I had lost the weight.

For 45 years I tried to live by Weight Watcher's weight loss program and it worked for me . . .for a while. I would usually let myself get about ten pounds over my healthy weight and re-up at the local WW meeting place, the

Methodist Church up on the hill. I'd lose the ten pounds after a couple months of weekly meetings, careful weighing of food, accountant-like focus on calorie tallying and religious exercise. Then as time drifted by, my resolve would gradually dissolve and I'd quit paying attention. Over time, usually about five years, I'd put my foot down and go back to WW, up ten pounds plus a few more.

By the time I was 50, I was returning to WW with 20 pounds to lose. At 65 I had not been to WW in seven years and I had 35 pounds to lose!

I've always had a stubborn streak but it takes more than stubbornness to stick to a Weight Watcher life-style for life, and I couldn't do it. But I'm not alone, I've watched WW leaders (including Jean Nidetch the founder) roller coaster their weight. Kirstie Alley couldn't do it. Oprah couldn't do it. I have many friends who couldn't do it. How's that Weight Watcher diet doing for you? You probably wouldn't be reading this book if it were working.

I was 68 years old when I found out why the Weight Watchers calories-in/calories-out theory does not work over time. It all has to do with what it considers a healthy diet. When I wrote *The Mouth Trap: the butt stops here!* I followed Weight Watchers guidelines, from portion control to going along with WW's food recommendations, along with major behavioral changes I'll tell you about later. I was as loyal to Weight Watchers as a student is to his mentor when it came to believing it was right. Now I know it's all wrong! You'll see as you read on, why very few of us can stay with a Weight Watcher's calories-in/calories out lifestyle.

Marla Cilley is who had sent *Why We Get Fat* to me. She had really embraced The Mouth Trap and I wondered why she'd sent this to me. Then, I read it! The first few chapters went exactly against everything I've ever believed about dieting. As I said, I always went to Weight

Watchers whenever I wanted to lose weight. Weight Watchers is built on a *supposed* "balanced" low fat, high carbohydrate diet recommended by the *supposed* health experts and medical community. As you will find out in my book, I went by that theory and diet plan to lose the weight. It works if you want to live a life always hungry and increasing your amount of exercise and decreasing your calorie intake as you get older. (I'll explain later by paraphrasing Gary's words.)

I couldn't put the book down! When I was finished with it I gave it to Terry to read, saying I was going to totally change the way I ate and I hoped he would too. Terry is a very skeptical person and being a journalist by trade, he wants all the facts void of emotion. He read the book in a couple of days and when he said he'd go along with me on changing our diet (and lifestyle as far as eating was concerned) I was so excited! Nelly was very quiet.

THE CHANGE

Gary's research is absolutely flawless! The way he presented research over the last 80 years is compelling and I would challenge anyone to find his opinion or emotion between the pages of *Why We Get Fat and What To Do About it*. I want you to read his book so you can be comfortable about the science that backs up his findings. Did you know that high cholesterol is not a determiner of heart disease and that there is no scientific proof that it is? Did you know that animal fat is not only extremely good for you, it's essential for healthy brain function? Did you know that fat doesn't make you fat? Did you know that the epidemic of auto-immune diseases is caused by the diet we've been told by our health experts and government is healthy?

Unlike Gary Taube's book, this book is filled with emotion and opinion as I tell you what has happened to Terry and me in the year that we've been on a restricted carbohydrate, high fat diet and lifestyle. I'm going to share with you my unscientific thoughts as a result of just living for more than a year of pure joy and extreme energy and well-being with this new way to eat.

What we learned from Gary's book in that first week in May 2011 was that carbohydrates (sugars, starches, grains) are what make us fat. They make us fat because they spike our insulin levels and our beautiful bodies don't know what to make of that so they go into what I've termed STUNTS mode. (Survival Threatened Urgent Need To Stockpile). In other words when you eat carbohydrates your body thinks it's in trouble (which it is) and it goes into survival mode.

What is a restricted carbohydrate diet? The number of carbohydrates you can healthfully consume daily is an individual matter that you will need to figure out for yourself. (It's somewhere between five and 100 grams of carbohydrates.) I have discovered I can have no more than 20 carbs a day. Terry can have 50. Today's medical wisdom (if you can call it that) insists that 300 grams of carbs a day is healthy! Unlike Gary Taubes I get to speak my mind on this. 300 carbs a day is insane. The medical experts have their heads up their assets to tell us we should consume 300 carbs a day. I don't think they are guilty of pre-meditated murder but certainly it's manslaughter. I know some nice doctors and I'm sure they haven't purposely told us to eat wrong so they have work, but that is exactly what they've done. And boy do they have work! Have you seen the statistics! There's an epidemic of diabetes, metabolic syndrome, Alzheimer's and Parkinson's Disease, MS, Cancer and obesity. How is that physician induced diet doing for us? We have been victims of this physician induced eating disorder and we don't have to be. People are sick because they've been told to eat wrong. We've been told what's wrong to eat for so long that what's right to eat sounds wrong. Read this next paragraph and see if your mind goes a little wonky.

Eat the skin on chicken, the fat on your steak, pork, lamb and fish, as many eggs as you want, butter, sour cream, mayonnaise, cheese, and stay away from anything with the word low cal or low fat on its label. Cook with lard and don't eat grains. How does that sound to you? Using my body as a lab for over a year, that's what I've adhered to every day and I've never been happier or healthier.

Unless you are blessed to already have an enlightened doctor who advocates a restricted carbohydrate/high fat diet, make it a priority to find one in your area who can support you in this major decision you'll be making. Jimmy Moore is an excellent resource and it was through his website www.livinlavidalowcarb.com that I was able to find Dr. Ann Childers in Portland, Oregon. Ann is also a psychiatrist who has expanded her medical practice to include helping people like me who want to be encouraged by a medical expert when going against the authority of our government and what they tell us we should eat, to most of the men and women in white coats with stethoscopes slung over their shoulders who are ignorant of the science and too arrogant to learn the truth and admit they've goofed BIG TIME.

I remember when I made my first appointment with Dr. Childers. I told her that I belonged to Kaiser (an HMO) and my physician (I'll call him Dr. Wrong) was a low-fat-three-eggs-a-week (and then only the whites) high-carbohydrate-type-guy and I wanted her to be my low-carb-two-eggs-a-day-skin-on-my-chicken doctor. I added that I was so angry with doctors who push the low fat, high carbohydrate diet and pills to lower cholesterol, that I just might need her as a shrink for anger management issues! (Sometimes I've come real close to needing her psychiatrically.) Embarking on this lifestyle, I took my health and life into my own hands and I thumbed my nose at Dr. Wrong's opinion of my restricted carbohydrate, high fat diet. It takes courage to go against authority and I'll be ever indebted to Dr. Childers for helping me make the leap.

One of the assignments Dr. Childers suggested at that very first appointment was to watch a documentary by Tom Naughton called *Fat Head*. Tom is a brilliantly funny writer and stars in the film. Terry and I watched it in that first month on our low-carb journey and could see why the good doctor insisted we see it. Tom not only explains for us non-science people what our bodies do with carbohydrates, he documents how we've been fed such a load of bologna by our government and our medical authorities. It is absolutely a must-watch and you'll see that I've put it into my assignment for this chapter.

After my first appointment with Ann, I felt such great relief and confidence that Terry and I were on the right path. She ordered blood work and also recommended I have a VAP cholesterol test which not only shows HDL and LDL, but shows the particle size of LDL which the standard, run-of-the-mill cholesterol test does not. Since I pay a lot of money to Kaiser for my health care ($400 a month) I decided to contact Dr. Wrong to at least get the tests done at Kaiser.

I emailed him and said, "Dear Dr. Wrong, I am currently seeing a psychiatrist outside of Kaiser, for an eating disorder." (I know I wasn't being totally honest, but Nelly loved having the slight stretch of the truth; and besides I did have an eating disorder—it just happened to be physician induced.) I went on to say in the email, "My psychiatrist has ordered some blood work and a special cholesterol test that's not the standard one Kaiser does. It's called a VAP test."

Dr. Wrong ordered the blood work, but questioned the VAP test. His email to me said, "I'm vaguely familiar with the VAP test, but I'm questioning why your psychiatrist wants this test, so I won't order it."

I answered, "Do you mean to tell me, unless you know my psychiatrist's motive, you won't order the test? If I have to go outside Kaiser for it, the cost to me will be $107!"

His answer, "Yes, I won't order it."

This is the arrogance we face with doctors who somehow come to think that MD stands for Minor Deity. (This was probably the closest I've come to needing Dr. Childers as a psychiatrist on my low carb journey.) But I really wasn't surprised at Wrong's response. For me it was just another sign I was on my own in this.

I did have the VAP blood test and the results brought rave reviews from Dr. Childers. If I hadn't had it I would not have known that my raised LDL count consisted of innocuous, fluffy particles as opposed to the dense particles that cause inflammation and can cause heart disease. There is another blood test called the NMR Lipoprofile, and Dr. Childers recommended I take this one because it is the most convincing lipid study in terms of LDL and whether it is likely to promote cardiovascular disease. I will have the test, but I don't see it as a big priority especially after reading a letter Rodney A. Hayward, MD and Harlan M. Krumholz, MD, from Yale wrote to the National Heart, Lung, and Blood Institute (NHLBI). "We are writing to encourage you to abandon the paradigm of treating patients to LDL targets, a change that will better align ATP IV(Adult Treatment Panel) with current clinical evidence. Changing long-held beliefs is never easy, even when the need for change is based on strong evidence. Change is especially difficult when prior beliefs are firmly embedded in culture, accepted as dogma, and codified in books, articles, guidelines, public service announcements, and performance measures."

As I wrote that last chapter, I felt as if there were an elephant in the room, so I'm going to address it. The elephant's name is Cholesterol. This elephant is no more a marker for heart disease than red hair is. Let me explain in very unscientific terms.

When you read Gary Taubes' book, *Why We Get Fat and What to do About it*, you'll find out that just as many people have heart attacks with low cholesterol as those with high cholesterol, NO DIFFERENCE. No studies have ever proven otherwise. Somehow (and you'll find out how in the book) we've been lead to believe we have to lower our cholesterol to avoid heart disease, and get this, at that same time drug companies came up with a drug that lowers cholesterol (they're called statins). Why would we take a cholesterol lowering drug if our cholesterol doesn't need to be lowered? We wouldn't. Somebody had to get us to think we needed to take it so they could push the drug. It's that simple! And push it they certainly do; to the tune of two billion dollars a year!

It would be like a company that makes red hair dye and wants to sell billions of bottles of it, so it starts a rumor that red heads don't have heart disease, so buy our dye and you won't die. Then they take out expensive ads in big deal medical journals and persuade doctors to recommend (prescribe) the dye to their patients, promising more ads if the physicians keep creating a demand. The red dye will no more prevent heart disease than the cholesterol lowering drugs will and yet most physicians prescribe them liberally.

I was one of those victims. After I read Gary's book I dumped my statins just like I did hormone therapy drugs way before it became public knowledge they caused breast cancer and heart attacks! If you are currently taking a statin, please don't dump them just because I did. Do your research and tell your low carb doctor what you want to do. Whatever you do, don't get into a big argument with the doctor who has prescribed them to you. You don't want to run up your blood pressure!

Just an aside, when I told Dr. Wrong via his nurse when I called to cancel a pap test (I don't have any more pap left to test) that I no longer take statins I stirred up a big fuss! I got a call from Wrong's PA (physician's assistant) Wrong Too asking me why I quit them statins. I told him no woman over 50 should be taking statins and if he didn't know that he was living in the dark ages. That didn't go over well with him. He also did not like hearing how healthy I am and kept acting like I was an exception to the rule. I ended up telling him to just write in my records "patient refuses prescribed drug" so he and Dr. Wrong can be off the hook for not making another sale.

Having to deal with a prejudiced physician is a waste of your time, money and health. Over the years it has cost me more money than I care to calculate and of course the good health I could have been enjoying. I'm very angry about this, because the truth has been known for a long time and it has been covered up.

One other thing about the elephant; we need Cholesterol and the older we get (especially women) our cholesterol should naturally go up. Over the last 40 years our population is getting fatter and fatter and sicker and sicker because we are starving our bodies by trying to follow what we've been told is a healthy diet. When we take our health into our own hands and back it up with help from a low carb doctor and lots of study on this subject, we can turn things around one body at a time.

Here's what has happened to my body in just 15 months into my new lifestyle.

- No achiness (The achiness quit when I quit taking the statins. I had thought all along the achiness was just old-lady pains.)

- The pockets in my gums closed up (When you get older your gums can begin to recede and my dentist measures the depth of the recession to determine whether treatment is necessary to stop the recession. My last exam revealed my gums have not only stopped receding, they've repaired themselves. My dentist was blown away and asked me what I'd been doing differently. I told him I was on a high fat, restricted carbohydrate diet that must have given my body the fuel it needed to heal itself.)

- Increased well-being

- Eczema disappeared and hasn't returned seasonally

- No sensitivity to heat (I used to be extremely sensitive to heat and had real problems in the summer and on vacation in the tropics. Not anymore!)

- Regular bowel movements (I used to have a bowel movement every three or four days).

- Energy level high (I never need a nap and I used to require one every day.)

- Nails are considerably stronger

- Triglycerides (one of the real markers for heart disease) have plunged from 155 to 62

- Weight loss and maintenance (My weight no longer fluctuates.)

- Never hungry

- A growth in my left hand dissolved

- Down four dress sizes

- No more bladder infections (I used to have two or three a year and was told by Dr. Wrong to stop taking baths and swimming in pools. Today I enjoy baths and swimming in pools.)

- Have not had a cold or flu (I didn't have a flu shot this year and in the past I averaged five colds a year.)

When I made this list it struck me that this lifestyle has literally slashed my need for medical services! Wow, what would happen if we all could cut out most of the need for them! I'll bet we wouldn't be hassling over healthcare issues because most of us would be healthy.

If I've convinced you that living a low-carb lifestyle is what you want to do, you'll want to start cooking low-carb. On my website www.makeitfunanditwillgetdone.com I have a low-carb cooking video segment every Monday. All of my low-carb recipes are archived on the website, just click on the Recipe tab. As I play in my kitchen and experiment with slashing carbs while still making tasty meals, I will continue to share my latest recipes.

Also on the website, you can watch top experts, doctors and researchers in the field of carbohydrate restriction. While on a low-carb cruise organized by Jimmy Moore and his fantastic staff, we listened to these men and women share their wisdom and knowledge with those of us who paid to go on the cruise with them and they were so gracious in allowing us to film their speeches for you, for free. Just go on the website and click on the Lose Weight tab.

Assignment for Chapter Two:

Watch *Fat Head* the documentary by Tom Naughton.

Read *Why We Get Fat and What do to About it* by Gary Taubes, before you embark on this path.

Chapter Three:
The End of a Love Affair (Sniff)

May 2009

Throughout my lifetime I'd had an on-going, dysfunctional, love affair with fat. For most of my adult life, my lover left me, came back, left, came back, left and came back. As I said earlier, I'd always turned to Weight Watchers for counsel. In fact, I'd joined seven times to get myself back in shape.

Looking back, each time that I returned for help I had a good reason: class reunions, my kids' weddings, and my second marriage. But, this time, I'd run out of good reasons to lose the thirty-five pounds I'd saved up. There was no class reunion coming up, no bathing suit vacation trip in the future that could have bolstered my resolve. Certainly, my doctor's advice to lower my cholesterol and high blood pressure by eating a low-fat, high carbohydrate diet and exercise more, didn't do it. I'd need to have the doctor say, "You're going to die in a week if you don't lose weight!" to get me motivated.

Reasonless and content for almost a year and moving day-by-day, ounce-by-ounce and inch-by-inch into the next size, I was accidentally struck with an incredible reason to end the love affair with my fat! While cleaning out a kitchen cupboard, I discovered an outdated five-pound sack of Gold Medal flour. I set it on the counter and finished cleaning the cupboard. Then I picked up the sack and headed for the garbage can when I thought, *Wow, five pounds is sort of heavy!*

I stopped, turned around and took the sack back into the kitchen. Then I thought to myself, *Let's walk around with it for 15 minutes to see how we feel.* It sounded like a good idea, so I carried it around the kitchen, into the living room, bedroom, bathroom, down to my office in the basement, back up the stairs and I still had ten more minutes! So, I strolled to the end of my drive-way (300 feet) and moseyed through my front yard and back down the drive-way again. When the 15 minutes was finally over, I was worn out from the burden of the extra weight. Then it hit me! I have SEVEN sacks of flour to lose!

The thought of carrying around seven of those sacks was suddenly and absolutely absurd! In essence I had been running a trucking company. Hello! I was 66-years-old and I didn't want to be bothered with losing and gaining, losing and gaining seven sacks of flour or more for whatever amount of time I had left! Right then and there I decided to be seven sacks lighter through my golden (not my Gold Medal) years! The blessing of the event was that I wholeheartedly grasped the idea of what I was doing to myself.

One of my on-line friends, Linnea, wrote me, telling of a similar story about her husband.

> *Lee found a beautiful rock a couple miles up the trail - it sparkled all over with encrusted crystals of Fool's Gold. He had to have it. Carrying it back was nearly impossible, it was so heavy. He arrived at the trail head exhausted and in pain. Later at home, he weighed it - 47 pounds. A light bulb moment - "I'm that much overweight - what would it be like to not carry that around?" A year later, he was 50 lbs. lighter and has kept it off for five years! The rock is on permanent display in a lighted alcove, where he has to pass it on the way to the pantry.*
> *Linnea*

"What would it be like to NOT carry that around?" I asked myself this same question, and then I went to Safeway and purchased seven five-pound bags of Gold

Medal flour (I dumped the outdated sack) and placed them in a prominent place on my kitchen counter. They were in my face during cooking and in my face during clean-up (two events that were major sources of unconscious nibbling). As I lost each five pounds I'd donate one of the sacks to the local food bank. I found other uses for them and I'll tell you about those in Chapter Five: *Your Very Own Rules.*

The eye-opening moments Lee, Linnea's husband and I experienced cut through denial and went straight to the heart of the matter. One of the many defenses an alcoholic uses is denial. Overeaters invariable use it too. Denial just means you aren't facing the truth. Denial is what kept me from enjoying the healthy happy weight I am today. The fact that I was in denial was a shock to me. I was denying I was in denial! Once I got past that hurdle, I discovered my denial was in layers that had to be peeled off at various intervals in order to get to the next layer. That's what takes time.

It was soon after my Gold Medal discovery that I came up with what I call the Wake-Up Collar. I took a pair of long pants (you could use pajama bottoms) and I tied a knot in each leg at the ankle.

I put one five-pound sack of flour down each leg so I was able to put the contraption around my neck. I decided I would wear it 15 minutes before each meal to remind me of my original reason to lose the weight and to stay out of denial. It really makes an impression on a child.

The Cruise Ship Behavior

As you cruise along on your voyage to lose your sacks of flour think about this. If the captain of a cruise ship wants to turn around and go in the opposite direction, the turnaround will take more energy, thought and action than just cruising forward in the same direction. Once he or she gets the ship going in the other direction then there is not as much to do except watch for stuff in the water.

Your ship (we'll call it the SS Behavior) needs to change its direction since you've decided to change your eating habits from the ones that put on the sacks to ones that take them off and eventually keep them off for the rest of your life. You are like the captain of the SS Behavior. In turning it around you have to be pre-occupied with your food and the eating of it. Until you've totally changed the direction of your thought the SS Behavior will keep going in the wrong direction. It takes time to turn a ship around!

We don't want these problems to take so much time! We've been raised on instant mashed potatoes. You will never see a headline like this on the cover of McCall's Magazine: *Bathing Suit Body by June 2017!!* Or *Get in Shape in Just One Year!* Or *From Kitchen to Table in Two Hour!* Our emphasis on taking our time and being kind and loving, but firm and persistent, is the key to our success.

If I was in denial, there's a good chance you are too. I'm going to help you bust through that denial so you can be free of its wicked consequences. You deserve to have a beautiful body that is healthy and happy. Let me repeat that. You deserve to have a beautiful body that is healthy and happy! Today is a new day.

How Denial and Ignorance Kept Me Caged in Fat

My body has very good proportion. Thank you, God. That has been a blessing and a curse. When I gain weight, it goes on evenly kind of like I've been dipped in wax. I can easily gain 15 pounds and stay in the same size albeit uncomfortably. When I lose weight, the same thing happens; it takes losing about fifteen pounds before anyone (including my husband) notices. Gradual weight-gain on a well-proportioned body is like having a kitchen floor that doesn't show dirt. It looks okay, but it's not healthy.

Looking back over my life I realized I'd gained ten pounds each decade. When I was 20-years-old I weighed 120 pounds and at 60, I weighed 160. By the time I got my first social security check I weighted 165. That's a gradual gain of one pound a year. Even a couple pounds a year doesn't sound like much, but in ten years if you don't change what you eat, you'll be lugging around an extra four sacks of flour. Add ten more years at that rate and you'll be at eight sacks of baggage! You can only dip an old lady in wax so many times before there's no denying there's a problem. One of the reasons old people get fat is we have time on our sides. In other words it's time that builds up the fat on our sides. The older we get the more time we have to add *just a little more*. And now I know it can all be blamed on carbohydrates.

It's a real challenge for me not be angry at those who have shoved a diet down our throats for forty year that is not only not healthy, but has damaged our health. If I'd only known back when I was 35 that carbohydrates were what caused me to gain, I wouldn't have ended up with that dipped in wax look, high blood pressure and a list of chronic troubles.

A Note on Exercise

It's a lot easier to NOT eat 500 calories a day (that's 50 McDonald's French fries and a Coke all carbs) than it is to walk for two hours up and down a mountain to burn 500 calories. It's the same 500 calories, whether you burned it by swimming or didn't consume it by escaping the drive-thru at the double arches. Don't expect exercise to cause drastic weight loss. Decide that you are going to exercise because it's good for your body, because it increases your metabolism, improves circulation, gives you a better night's sleep, improves your physical and mental health, improves your physical appearance, strength and mobility, and because it makes you feel great.

Get exercise for the right reasons, those I just mentioned. Otherwise you'll be disappointed at how little effect it can have on your total weight loss. For one thing, muscle weighs more than fat. As you begin to get rid of the fat and build muscle, your great efforts can look like weight gain! It's true that exercise builds muscle and muscle burns fat, but your scale doesn't know the difference. It just weighs what's put on it. I read somewhere that a pound of fat is about the size of a cantaloupe, and a pound of muscle is about the size of a peach. By all means, exercise every day, but don't get discouraged if your scale tries to tell you that your effort to lose weight is not working.

It occurred to me about a year on our low-carb lifestyle that if I were using the calories-in-calories-out theory, I should weigh 288 pounds today! I figured it out as Terry and I were waiting for our lunch in a restaurant in Cancun, Mexico.
Going to Cancun was a little scary because the food is full of carbohydrates. Tacos, burritos, tamales, quesadillas, margaritas and tortillas! What was a low carb couple to do in Mexico for two whole weeks?

We'd been a year into our low-carb lifestyle and we were curious as to how we would navigate our way around the temptations of Mexican treats like refried beans, rice and tortilla chips.

The hardest part was seeing fellow diners enjoying baskets of hot corn chips with fresh salsa while we'd sit rearranging our silverware, small talking over glasses of ice water and fishing out the wedges of lime for another squeeze in wait for our meals.

The second hardest part was watching those chip eating, margarita drinking diners get served hamburgers with buns and piles of piping hot French fries accompanied by a big bottle of ketchup (all no nos on a low-carb lifestyle).

Those psychological hurdles were over and we were home free once our healthy choices of fish, cheese, beef, chicken, shrimp or lobster came wafting to our table, served with extra butter and guacamole.

It was one week into the vacation as we were eating our high fat, low carb lunches on a terrace of one of our many favorite restaurants that a profound notion hit me! I have to warn you, this is going to have good news as well as bad news in it.

The AHA moment came with the realization that I am scientific proof that the "calories-in-calories-out" theory of weight loss is critically flawed! With the help of Terry's left-brain, we concluded that since we started our new way to eat, I should weigh 143 pounds more than I do right now! That means I'd weigh 288 pounds!

Here's why: I used to walk five miles a day, six days a week, up 1,100 feet in elevation. It took me approximately one hour and 45 minutes and I burned approximately 500 calories. But since we'd gone low-carb I had quit walking. Sitting at that table in Cancun we figured in one year I hadn't taken 288 walks. That worked out to be 144,000 calories I didn't burn. Divided by 3,500 (that's how many calories there are in a pound) we figured I should have gained 41 pounds.

Then we figured I'm eating about 1000 calories more a day than I was before May 2, 2011 which should have added an additional 102 pounds. In fact I weigh 10 pounds less than I weighed on May 2.

So where did all those calories go? I know they didn't go on my hips and thighs. Since my hair is shinier, my skin is moister and my energy level is higher, I believe they went to repair cells, build tissue, fight off germs, and take care of my body as it has never been taken care of before. I believe I had been starving my body of the essential food it has needed for more than 50 years and now it's celebrating my new diet.

I have started walking again, but I'm not going five miles six days a week. Instead I walk 45 minutes four days and let my body rest the other three.

Watch For Shifts in Attitude and Behavior

As I progressed, I began to focus more on my attitude and behavior and less on my weight. I noticed a huge shift one weekend, about three months into my program. We were hosting a party for our neighbors at our home. Here in the foothills of the Cascade Mountains, our homes are far apart from each other. Despite the distance and even though we rarely see one another, we have an annual "hill" party. 30 families came to our house for a potluck of salads and desserts. We provided barbecued ribs and chicken, beverages and hors d'oeuvres. As the salads arrived, I kept eyeing them. I didn't pay much attention at first but after a while I realized I was more interested in the salads than the desserts. When did that happen? The change was gradual because it happened in my head, just as gradual as the changes in our bodies as we lose weight. Be watching for those priceless shifts in thinking as you journey ahead.

One of my neighbors, whom I hadn't seen in a year, commented on my weight-loss.

"How did you do it?" She had a piece of apple pie, a lemon tart and homemade almond candy on her plate.

"Well, for one thing, I realized that I was equating fun with food," I said. We were chatting by a tray of fresh, colorful red, orange and green peppers I'd cut up for hors d'oeuvres.

"Fun, with food?"

"Yeah! Take these veggies for instance, can you look at them and think fun?"

"No! They're *pretty*, but they're not fun! This," she held up her plate, "this is fun!"

That notion is classic. We equate sugary foods with fun. That's because many of the sugary foods we love are associated with celebrations and feasts! Parties! Weddings! Holidays! Happy Hours! Taking a bite of food has nothing to do with fun unless you choose to make that connection. What appears to be fun is only happening in your mind.

About a year ago I invited a neighbor to walk with me. She said she would after the first of the year. At the time, she told me her downfall was M & M candies. Did you know one M & M is 4.3 calories? That means that a handful (average 10) of those seemingly innocuous little critters is 43 calories. If you passed the M & M candy bowl three times a day and scooped up a little handful, in a year you would gain 12 pounds on M & Ms alone. I saw my neighbor at the store recently and I'm sure she is testimony to my calculation. If M & Ms are your downfall (or whatever you say is) see them as clothes fitting too tightly, struggling to move, heart constricting arteries, cancerous tumors, or diabetes. In other words picture the consequences before you consider eating something.

Speaking of M & Ms, here is an aside on the subject of your sweet tooth, if you have one. I've thought a great deal about our love of sweet tasting foods and why we do love them. Then I remembered being a new mother and wondering what breast milk tasted like. I had to taste it, as disgusting as the thought was to me at the time. If you've tasted human breast milk then you know what I'm going to tell you. I was shocked by how sweet it was. To me it was sweeter than if I put a cup of sugar in two cups of cow's milk. I think there is a link between our first food and what we end up wanting when we are adults.

Taste can be a trained response as can your notions about food, but reprogramming your thinking takes time and anything that takes time takes patience. When you achieve your goal, you will be glad you learned to be patient with yourself.

Elaine, a person I've shared my journey with, told me she now has a different way of looking at the foods she once viewed as "fun."

> *Yesterday my husband and I went out for dinner. I ate salmon, green beans and strawberries. What didn't I eat? Well, there was that cellulite that was served in the form of long pasta noodles with tomatoes and oregano from the garden, and the heart attack that was a dinner-sized plate of strawberry shortcake, strawberry ice cream and low fat whipped topping (as if that would redeem anything!). When I got home there was the belly ache I avoided by not eating the bag of red licorice that someone had kindly left on the table to share.*

That notion is classic. We equate sugary foods with fun. That's because many of the sugary foods we love are associated with celebrations and feasts! Parties! Weddings! Holidays! Happy Hours! Taking a bite of food has nothing to do with fun unless you choose to make that connection. What appears to be fun is only happening in your mind.

Start looking at your food with new eyes. Instead of smelling the aroma of the Cinnabon in the air and following your nose to a moist, sugary fun-filled cinnamon roll like a basset hound, sniff the air like Bambi's mother did when she smelled the hunters and run the other way! My new eyes took time to adjust to and I definitely developed patience.

If you've ever been in a relationship that didn't work out, you know you didn't just say, "Well, that affair is over, we were in love but oh well."

No, there was a period of grieving. You pined, phoned and hung up and saw others who reminded you of your ex. You cried, sniveled, whined and cried some more. Constant reminders plagued you. Certain music, the time of day, that chair, that car... You schemed for ways to reconcile.

Finally it sunk in and you got it; it was over! Recognizing it was over didn't mean you weren't still grieving. You were still sad that the love affair ended. Only time and new love can heal the loss completely.

My dear, that love affair is food high in carbohydrates. That love affair is the combination of friends, tradition and maybe addiction. That love affair is the notion that fun means food. And now it's over and it IS sad. Boo hoo, now you have to make new friends (meats (not lean), eggs, nuts, cheese, mayonnaise, sour cream, butter, high fat yogurt, vegetables, water), find new activities (less television and computer time), new places that don't remind you of your old love affair (no more fast food) and a new meaning for fun.

Experts say grieving is a process. It's a process whether you've lost a foot, a fellow or the food you loved. It takes as much as a year to go through all the stages of grief for most people. Occasions such as birthday parties, barbeques, pot lucks, holidays, anniversaries, vacations and the like will feel different after the loss. Just remember, if you are like most people it'll be a year before you are completely comfortable with the new you.

Deciding to make changes in your eating habits is the easy part. It's easy to say, "I'm going to lose five sacks of flour this year." Actually doing it requires your undivided attention when you are around food. We are all creatures of habit and we fall into routines that serve us well or - not so well. Up until now your eating routine has burdened you with quite a few bags of flour. When you make something a habit (good or bad) you don't have to pay so much attention to what you are doing. That's how you can eat a cupcake and not remember you ate it.

We are masters at "getting used to things," otherwise we wouldn't be able to get used to dragging around an extra sack of flour let alone five, ten or more of them. The fact that we do get used to things is good news! It means that as we re-program a thought such as, 'Yippee, the party is tonight. I wonder what the food will be,' to a thought such as: 'Yippee, the party is tonight, I wonder who will be there?' it will become a habitual response.

At first the thought will be foreign and you'll have to deliberately hardwire it in as the new default thought concerning all social affairs. With practice and patience you will gradually change the priority you've put on food from "I get to eat" to "I have to eat." Also, the realization of how much work is involved in chewing a meal properly will help you see food with new eyes.

Thin people don't think about food. My friend Marion is very thin and once she said, "I don't get it. Why do people have to talk about food all the time? Why do we have to go out to lunch? How come we can't catch up on a walk?" I've heard Marion say, "I forgot to eat!" She's free! She eats because she has to, not because she's been counting down the minutes until the next feeding.

Right now you're probably preoccupied with food (like you would be if you just broke up with your lover) because you've decided to lose weight. That's normal. But as you move slowly toward your goal weight you will notice a gradual shift in your priorities. You'll notice that food won't be one of those priorities. In time, you won't be preoccupied with food even when you are really hungry. You'll think, "Oh I have to eat something," not "I'm STARVING."

The unknown is scary! The truth, of course, is that change can be a wonderful gift. In fact, it is the key that unlocks the doors to growth and excitement. That's because when you change habitual thinking into new thoughts, your emotions get to come out and play. When old patterns are broken, new worlds emerge.

As you begin this journey remember your new reason to do this. You are sick and tired of hauling around the flour sacks. (Hopefully you are going to put at least one on your kitchen counter.) Making the break with your old love affair will be as easy or as difficult as you decide it's going to be. Decide right now, before you go on to Chapter Four, that you are going to start changing that magical mind of yours today and you have a whole year to re-program it.

When initially I gave myself a whole year to get over the affair, I learned such valuable lessons. One came right after the holidays. I'd been sailing along for eight months, enjoying the loss of four sacks of flour, getting used to how much easier it was to exercise, taking glee in tossing winter clothes I'd pulled out of storage that were way too big and getting compliments from various friends and relatives who had noticed I'd lost a little.

With the onslaught of the holidays, beginning with Thanksgiving and ending with a New Year's Eve party I gained five pounds! I thought I was over the love affair, but it was really like the song from the 40s, That Old Feeling:

> I saw you last night and got that old feeling
> When you came in sight I got that old feeling
> There'll be no new romance for me
> It's foolish to start
> For that old feeling is still in my heart

What was positive about the holiday experience was that I was kind to myself in spite of the weight gain. I chalked it up to learning that I wasn't quite over my love affair. But almost! The holidays take up almost seven weeks out of a year. If you're entertaining and being entertained it's easy pack on a sack of flour, especially if alcohol is served. Remember; "It's hard to lose if you drink too much booze."

Assignment for Chapter Three:

Weigh yourself on a good scale. If you don't have a good scale, get one. (Not weighing once a week is like not balancing your checkbook regularly.) Buy the equivalent weight you want to lose, in five whatevers. Since I've eliminated flour and sugar from our diet I can't tell you to go buy it, because that's what I did before I knew how horrible it is for us. I suggest finding bricks that weigh five pounds or as one person suggested five pound sacks of coffee or nuts. Place those five pound whatevers throughout your home as a constant reminder of your goal. Self-discipline is remembering what you REALLY want. With these reminders in strategic places you will not only be reminded of what you REALLY want, you will smile.

Write a couple paragraphs (in present tense) on how you envision yourself a year from now. Write about how you look, how you feel, how other people see you, what things you will be able to do that you can't do now. Print it out and put it where you can see it every day. Read it every day.

Here is an example:

I love weighing what I weighed in high school, not only for the way I look, but how I feel moving around, playing with my kids, and how happy I am to have my husband tell me I'm sexy. I love the new clothes I had to buy because none of my old clothes fit anymore. It's fun to be in the newest fashion and wear the new colors on my body instead of always wearing black to hide my bulges. I love how I am not preoccupied with what I'm going to eat and I love knowing when I'm satisfied and never feeling stuffed. I am amazed at how young I look and how much more energy I have now that I'm the weight I was meant to be. I am so happy I look forward to my exercise and that it isn't something I wish I didn't have to do. I love playing my music and dancing and stretching. I am proud of myself and I love knowing myself better because of the weight I've lost.

Chapter Four

Enjoy!

We are supposed to enjoy our food, but most of us really don't. You're probably thinking, 'Wait a minute, I love food and I *do* enjoy it. That's the main reason why I'm overweight!'

Think about this. What do you like most about eating? Is it when the food hits your stomach? Is it the swallow and the texture of the food going down your throat? Or is your favorite part the aroma of good food and the taste while it's in your mouth? Your answer is probably the latter. We have been given such a gift in taste.

I'll bet God thought, *'Hmm, my little humans are going to have to eat several times a day and knowing how busy they'll get I'd better put some kind of an alarm in their brains to remind them it's time to eat again (I'll call it hunger), and I'll put a device in the hole I've made for the food to go in that will cause them to enjoy what they put in it.'* So He invented the tongue with buds all over it to enjoy the taste of sweet, salt, sour and bitter.

Then He designed the nose with two holes in it so we could breathe while we chew (since it should take about a minute of chewing per bite). Then I think He threw in the sense of smell mostly so we'd be able to enjoy a million other subtle tastes He created for us.

In all the years you've owned your mouth; you probably haven't paid that much attention to it. Sure you take care to brush your teeth after meals, to floss and to visit the dentist regularly.

You decorate the outside of your mouth with lipstick and use lip balm when your lips get chapped, but have you really paid attention to its *internal* workings? Awareness of what goes on in your mouth is the key. It's a mental matter.

By mindfully enjoying meals, for more than three years, I've examined and analyzed the "bite," as if I were a devoted researcher working with state of the art equipment. I've discovered some very important information that involves focused attention to the common bite of food we take. The result of my research will help you enjoy your food ten times more than you do now and ultimately lose weight because you'll be satisfied with less.

Our enjoyment of food lies in the taste, which is the tongue's job, along with its worthy partner the nose. As soon as you swallow, the duo is through working (except for sleuthing work by the tongue as it checks for stuff that's stuck in your teeth and hiding places in your mouth). So, once the food has left the room the pleasure goes with it. Think of a bite of food as if it were a comedian you love. If you invited that comedian to entertain at your party, you wouldn't have him come and tell one joke and leave. You'd want him to stay in the room and tell as many jokes as he could and the longer he could stay the better. Your tongue is like a person just waiting to be entertained. If you want to increase the pleasure of eating, don't swallow so fast. When you prolong the chewing process prior to the swallow and let your tongue play its impressive role in your enjoyment, you'll be getting the most out of eating. You'll be getting the biggest bang for your bite. You'll automatically take longer to eat and you'll eat less, because your stomach will have time to tell you it's full. Incidentally, the voice that tells you you're full is very, very quiet like the one you'd use in church to tell your husband his fly is unzipped. The voice that tells you you're hungry is loud and obnoxious like the one you'd use to tell him for the millionth time to PUT DOWN THE TOILET SEAT.

So let me ask you a question; how many times, just off the top of your head, do you think you chew each bite? I've observed that most people take a bite and chew about ten times. When I started "studying" my own chewing habit I discovered with one bite (about a tablespoon) I would chew 10 to 15 times, depending on the liquid content of the food, and my brain would *begin* to tell me "it's almost time to swallow." (I now know that was just a habit I'd gotten into because somewhere along the line, I'd gotten in a big hurry.)

If you REALLY want to expand the enjoyment of your food, don't swallow until you've chewed between 60 and 100 times! Remember, the longer you can keep a bite in your mouth, the longer you get to enjoy it. It's that simple.

All you need to do is intercept the message that it's almost time to swallow and instead store what's in your mouth into your cheeks for further processing (like chipmunks do) swallowing any liquid that has accumulated in there as you continue to chew. Ultimately you will turn one bite into several swallows (three to four) instead of just one.

I've been observing the miraculous work of my tongue for the last three years and have great respect for what it does in my mouth. It's an athlete and it has a very dangerous job! It can do things I never knew it could do until I really paid attention. For one thing, during a bite, your tongue is constantly moving the food back and forth in your mouth. It reminds me of a factory worker on an assembly line, conveying a product back and forth under treacherous grinders (our teeth are made of the hardest substance in our bodies for a good reason, they're meant to process food) kicking out foreign materials like seeds and fish bones. If you've ever bitten your tongue, you know what dangerous work it does! Bless its heart!

One more note while I'm talking about taking one bite. A marshmallow-sized bite is too big! Too much food in your mouth is like too many people in a room. What fun is that? Not one of us likes too big a crowd and neither does our tongue. Your tongue can get confused when it has to process too much food. You could even choke on too big a bite. If you've been guilty of taking big bites, you can start today to take smaller ones. And then take the time to enjoy each and every one.

The process of chewing is called mastication. It is almost a lost art, especially in our frenetic society. Today we use terms like scarf down, gobble up, pig out, gulp, guzzle and gorge to describe our dining experiences. Most people are unconscious masticators. To make mastication a conscious process is an art! As you practice, you'll become a skilled masticator and it will serve you well. I almost feel as if I have a degree in masticology. If you consider your mouth to be a food processor you can really have fun with this and be on your way to your own degree.

From now on when you are around other people, observe how many chews they take with each bite and you'll be amazed at how fast most people process their food (and how fast you've been processing yours).

Midway in my journey I was out one evening with the girls and as the five of us sat around a table enjoying pizza, I nonchalantly counted different women's chews per bite (it's easy to do without getting caught, especially when the gossip starts). True to my theory, the thin women in the group took small bites (about the size of a cherry) and chewed around 25 chews per bite. The one overweight woman was wolfing down apricot-size bites and averaging five chews to a swallow.

To get started becoming a master masticator, here's an important warm up exercise I recommend doing as soon as possible.

Broil a four ounce sirloin steak to your liking. Pour a tall glass of water and sit down to your meal. The steak should be around 20 bites. I recommend getting a little one-minute timer, you know the glass kind with sand in it. I extend my minute-per-bite ratio by putting God into a five-second pause before each bite. That adds a minute and a half to my meal. Do not use your water to "wash" down a swallow. Drink only when your mouth is empty. Let the natural secretions (spit) lubricate your swallow. For effective mastication you need natural lubrication. Ahemm.

While you eat, tally your bites and count your chews. Allot at least 60 chews per bite and pay attention to the miracle of your tongue. The first time I did this exercise I could honestly say I never enjoyed my food more. I remember my jaws were sore afterward and I couldn't finish the whole steak. I had to wrap it up and save it for later. Once you do this exercise you'll want to always eat that way and you'll never look at a piece of bacon or sirloin steak the same way! i.e.: It'll look yummy but it'll look like a lot of work!

When I shared my lunch experience with my husband that night, he wanted to try it with dinner. The first thing I noticed was we didn't talk much. We were too busy chewing and of course enjoying our food. Neither of us let one bite go unconscious and have for the most part become master masticators. I highly suggest doing this mindful eating *whenever* you're alone. As time goes on, you'll get better and better at staying aware when you're eating around others. It won't be long before you'll be able to eat without counting chews because you'll get used to feeling the consistency of what the food should be (like baby food) when you swallow it. Imagine that you are a blender and your mouth is set on "puree." Very soon you'll get to a place where you will never swallow hunks of unprocessed food again. Oh, and your stomach will thank you!

It's difficult to masticate in public and stay aware of the process. It takes practice to stay alert. You'll be surprised how many of your bites will be unconscious (therefore not enjoyed) even though you've planned to be vigilant. As you chat with your family or friends be mindful and catch yourself when you are sidetracked by someone's comments or your own thoughts and you miss the pleasure of what is in your mouth. If you tend to be an *emotional* eater, this experiment (ultimately a practice) will be enlightening.

If we're not careful, most of our eating is unconscious. We might enjoy that first bite of something but as the meal continues we get distracted and forget to enjoy even our favorite foods as the bites go on. Have you ever noticed when you are in a restaurant how a noisy table gets quiet when the food is served? That's because for the first few bites the eaters are paying attention to the food they put in their mouths. Invariably the noise level resumes as the eaters fall into unconscious mastication on about the fourth bite.

One of the main reasons we overeat is we forget to enjoy what we eat so we are left with that *is-that-all-there-is* feeling. Then we eat more, subconsciously hoping that feeling of enjoyment we're missing will somehow miraculously appear, only to go unconscious with the next bite and the next. We have to retrain ourselves to stay conscious and focus on each and every bite we take. Counting chews will help you become aware. It takes practice but it's very rewarding. What could be more fun than to practice enjoying *every* bite you take, and reduce your weight at the same time?

The Vicarious Bite

Another lesson I learned was my ability to enjoy a bite of food vicariously. If you are a dog owner you've no doubt experienced your dog drooling as he/she watched you eat something. I think the dog is drooling because it can imagine having your food in its mouth. If a dog can do this so can you.

Because you already know what a cinnamon roll tastes like (thank goodness for memory) you can remember and imagine what it tastes like. You can learn how to watch someone take a bite of something you'd like to eat and enjoy it almost as much as the person who is actually eating it. (When he/she has started unconsciously eating, after the first few bites you can actually enjoy the bites more that the eater does.) It takes practice and it's good to get permission from the eater you're going to use. Most likely you'll want to limit this exercise to friends and family. People generally don't like to be stared at, especially if you are drooling, but if you follow my method you'll put the eater at ease. Here's how it works.

You see the eater ready to enjoy a piece of homemade wild blackberry pie and you say,

"Excuse me, I can't have any pie but would you mind if I watched you while you eat yours?"

The eater will usually allow the audience. As you practice this mind game you'll get better at watching and you won't even have to ask. A sure sign you are getting good at this is when you have to swallow because the vision has made your mouth water.

If you are going to play with me I can promise you that for a while you're going to be preoccupied with food; what you eat, how much you eat, why you eat, where you eat, how many times you chew and when you eat. That preoccupation is normal and necessary for the changes you are going to make. After a while that preoccupation will leave and you'll have a new mindset when it comes to eating.

Once I was on my walk and I was very hungry so I took ten minutes while I kept walking and enjoyed a Whopper in my mind. (The beauty of eating in your mind is you don't have to chew. No work involved!)

Sue, an on-line friend of mine with whom I've shared many of my ideas for this book in order to get feedback, had some interesting observations on the topic of using imagination in this journey to a lighter life. She said, "I am becoming more and more aware of how susceptible I am to the influence of TV and how I let my mental perception of how something tastes merge with the images on the screen and create a desire to really experience it.

It's not just those expertly crafted food commercials either. I was watching the kid's TV show *Arthur* (which isn't even live action, it's *drawn* images!) and first they were eating popcorn (lumpy white circles) and I got up to get some! Later they were eating sundaes and I wanted one (fortunately we don't have any ice cream in the house). I wonder if an active imagination is a common link with overweight people. Is this how we get into trouble? We see someone eating and we think, 'That would taste good right now!' or 'Oh yeah, I used to love eating that! Mmmm, it tasted sooo good. I haven't eaten that in a while. Wonder if it still tastes the same?'

"I think you hit on something when you talked about hunger after 7 pm as fake hunger. You also called it habit hunger, but fake hunger is the perfect term! Why has no one ever called it that? It's not that my **digestive** system is empty; it's all in my **head**! And what am I frequently doing after 7 pm? I'm sitting in front of the TV! And get this; my favorite shows are on *The Food Network!!* Oh my goodness, what a light bulb moment! I started cutting back on my TV viewing and the night snacks have gone right out the window."

Thank you Sue!

Start enjoying your food more today! With the next bite you take, you have the power to stay conscious and enjoy that bite. A person I once knew had a little sign on his desk. All it said was "Think." He said that reminder had kept him from ever taking a drink. It was given to him by his sponsor at AA. In my journey, I've thought about that sign a lot. If we "think" we will enjoy!

Assignment for Chapter Four:

Arrange to be alone and eat your steak, following the directions given in this chapter.

Start observing others while they eat and keep remembering to enjoy what you have in your mouth.

Begin watching when a desire for a certain food pops up and ask four questions I will repeat several times in this book: Am I thirsty? Tired? Do I need some fresh air? Am I upset with a circumstance other than hunger?

Have fun!

Chapter Five:
Your Very Own Rules

I hope you are eager to move forward. In the chapter assignments, I've been giving you ideas for supplies. Here's a recap with a few other items I think will help you.

1. The equivalent number of five-pound "whatevers" representing the weight you want to stop lugging around.
2. A pair of long pants tied in a knot at the bottom of each leg, for your Wake Up Collar.
3. A month's worth of Weekly Progress Reports in a binder (instructions are later in this chapter).
4. A good scale.
5. A timer.
6. A small spiral notebook (such as a reporter's notebook) to take with you wherever you go.
7. A water bottle.
8. A carb counter. (You NEVER have to count calories again!)

Remember, my guidelines are not set in stone; they are merely springboards for you to take your own fertile imagination with on your journey. Feel free to try your own tweakings and testings of the rules I suggest here. Make up your own rules.

Here are the rules I made for Nelly and me.

Rule One:

If your doctor is closed minded and insists that a restricted carbohydrate, high fat diet is not healthy, find a low carb doctor who knows the truth about the science. The best source to find a physician near you is to go to Jimmy Moore's website www.livinlavidalowcarb.com. That's how I found Dr. Anne Childers in the Portland area. I am so thankful to have her as a physician and a friend. It's scary to go against authority of doctors, and if it were not for Dr. Childers I don't think I would have had the nerve to be so revolutionary.

Rule Two:

If you decide to follow a low carb, high fat diet start cleaning out your pantry of the foods that are high in carbohydrates. You'll be shocked at how high some foods are. For example: a glass of orange juice is 27 carbs and a piece of whole wheat bread is 26 carbs. I can only have 15 carbs a day so the bread and juice would be three days of carbs for me. Also dump all products that claim low fat, like low fat mayonnaise, cottage cheese, milk and so forth.

Rule Three:

Set a goal of losing one pound a week. Tell your inner child something like this: "We just have to lose five pounds and we're going to take five weeks to do that." If you are alone right now, repeat after me: "We just have to lose five pounds and we have five weeks to do that."

That's right. Let that idea soak right down into your bones. Just five pounds. The only difference between a person who just has five pounds to lose and one who has 75 pounds to lose is, the second person will be saying, "We just have to lose five pounds," *longer*.

Track the loss of the five pounds using the *Weekly Progress Reports*, which you will find on my website: www.makeitfunanditwillgetdone.com I suggest a goal of one pound a week because that is a safe and healthy amount. Remember, I lost 35 pounds in two years, gained ten back and lost the ten switching to the low carb lifestyle. Now that I'm low carb, my weight has stopped vacillating.

Notice I didn't give you a "time frame" for losing *all* the weight, just five pounds in five weeks. If you don't lose five pounds in five weeks, BIG DEAL! The most important thing is that you keep in touch with your inner child and stay on the program. Why not set an END deadline?

There are some valid reasons not to. I am a procrastinator and deadlines certainly do help me get things like writing books finished, but, on the other hand, when it comes to losing weight, setting the end deadline has backfired so many times because I proceeded to treat the completed goal just like a work deadline.

In other words: "There, now that's over with!"

Now if you embark on this program and you have some big deal event coming up like a class reunion, your wedding, or an audition for a movie role, you certainly can use the extra motivation to look good as momentum. The reason I have taken a deadline out of the equation is because I want you to focus on your behavior on a daily basis. The results of that new behavior—a happy, healthy body—will occur naturally.

Your inner child will go along with the program more easily when she realizes you're not going to beat her up for failing to meet some arbitrary end-of-the-road deadline. And finally when you do get to your goal you will NOT treat it like the project is over so now you can go back to the old behavior.

Rule Four:
Use a Weekly Progress Report every week

How to Use the Weekly Progress Report

In the space for "YOUR RULES" write what you will do to reach your weekly goal of losing one pound. Your rules might be, this week, I will not eat sugar, bread, potatoes, rice or pasta and I will walk two miles each day.

In the space for "REASONS" write the reasons your inner child will go along with your rules. In most cases your inner child will have very immature reasons for going along with the program. For example here are Nelly's reasons for going along with my rules of no sugar, bread, potatoes, pasta or rice and to walk five miles every day. She wants to act like a "smarty pants" around Gina, look cute and sexy like Sarah Rae and make the neighbor wish he could "stay over." Remember an inner child is between six and nine years old. Do you think a child could give a rip about the need to lower triglycerides or blood pressure? Of course not.

In the space for "REWARD," write down some way to pamper yourself.

The rest of the report is for the interaction you have with your inner child on a daily basis. There is a place to put the day and date and a place to give you and your inner child a grade (ABCD or F) three times each day. In the beginning you'll want to grade yourself in the morning, afternoon and evening. At the end of the week your grade will be an average of your daily grades.

In the beginning you will need to write all the excuses she will come up with, the flack she'll throw at you and the arguments you will have with her. You will be catching her trying to trick you into disobeying the rules. Don't forget, self-discipline is remembering what you REALLY want.

At the bottom of the report is a place for a final grade for the week.

Did you know that keeping a food diary can double a person's weight loss? It's true, according to a study conducted by Kaiser Permanente's Center for Health Research in Portland, Oregon. The report was published in the August 2008 edition of the *American Journal of Preventive Medicine*. One man who was part of the study had lost over 100 pounds. He said that the most difficult part of the experience was writing down every morsel of food that he ate, but he also said that was the reason he was successful. He would think twice about having that cookie because he didn't want to have to write it down and expose his lack of will power.

Until week sixteen of my program Nelly balked at keeping a journal of everything she ate. After a highly volatile confrontation (like nothing I'd seen in a couple of years) I told her we were going to start keeping a journal. It took some time, but I finally got to the bottom of her problem. Since we write for a living, the word *journal* ticked her off. I told her if the word was so distasteful, she should come up with another word for keeping track of everything she eats. About five hours later this was her response: A Consumer Report! Seems filling out a report isn't as daunting as writing in a journal. Whatever.

In those first two years when I was counting calories, I began keeping track in my notebook in a section called, Nelly's Consumer Report. I'll tell you more about it in Chapter Six. With her blessing, I bought a food scale so I could re-acquaint myself with weights of food and be able to make an accurate consumer report. The man in the Kaiser study was right; knowing exactly what you consume while you are losing weight is very important. After I dumped the Weight Watcher way of dieting and started my low-carb, high fat diet all I needed to do was keep track of carbs. It is so freeing never to count calories again, and since I can't have over 15 carbs a day, I only have to count to 15.

If you don't have a Consumer Report going, start one along with the Weekly Progress Report. One of the great benefits of filling out these reports is you are giving your inner child attention. Just remember your rules and your inner child's reasons. Nelly's ultimate reason for wanting to lose weight was that she's lazy and refuses to even consider carrying those sacks around ever again.

Rule Five:
Drink plenty of water.

Rule Six:
Make it fun and it will get done. Find ways to make this project fun! Terry and I went on a low-carb cruise with 300 other low-carbers and physicians, researchers and experts in the field and my birthday happened to fall while we were on the cruise. Since I don't eat cake I decided to have the waiters bring to our dinner table a big filet mignon decorated in butter with a candle in the middle. Everyone sang "Happy Birthday," and I cut the birthday steak into wedges and served the people at our table. Now that was fun.

Take your imagination as far as you can. One day about six months into my project I received an email from a woman named Suzanne. She wrote about her imaginary backpack. When I responded and thanked her for the idea, this is what she sent to me.

Thank you, Pam. I'm glad you like my little idea. I've been working on making it into a book, What Color Is Your Backpack? I work as a Special Ed. Aide and was using it with the kids at school. They'd rush to my desk first thing in the morning to tell me what color their backpack was and what they put in it for the day. As they got more creative, so did my Inner Child, Suzie Q. She started coming up with things I barely remembered playing with until she brought them vividly to mind.

In the Hawaiian religion they knew about the Inner Child for hundreds of years. They thought people had three parts. The Father or Higher Self who talks to God, The Mother, or regular consciousness, or what we think of as "us," and the Inner Child who is really the subconscious and has memories going back to the beginning of creation. And unless that Inner Child feels loved, and knows that we're sorry for any wrong doing we've committed, she won't let us appeal to God because we're unworthy. So the Hawaiians took care of the Inner Child with these four phrases: I'm Sorry, Forgive Me, Thank You, I Love You, then they would pray to God saying , Father, Mother, Child as one we ask . . .so that they were praying with all parts of themselves in alignment. The really cool thing is that the things you put in the backpack are there to keep her amused when she gets tired of cleaning up all the negative memories and connections that is her chief job. You just say "Clean, clean, erase, erase" and off she goes taking care of business.

I don't know if you ever read the article by Joe Vitale about Dr. Hew Len who cured an entire ward of criminally insane patients? He would lock himself in his office. The ward was so dangerous, even shackled; the inmates could and did hurt people. Dr. Len would study their files to see what in him could have caused their awful deeds to exist in his world. This was a system created by a Hawaiian Kuhuna named Mornnah Simeona who completely revamped an old Hawaiian system called Making Things Right or Ho'oponopono. Her solution was to take responsibility for everything. See an injustice? Get your little one busy cleaning and erasing it, clean, clean, erase, I'm Sorry, Forgive Me, Thank You, I Love You. Once the Inner Child was on your side, you could ask God to transmute any problem.

Well, I sure couldn't use the God part at a public school, but I could use the Inner Child, and Pam the way the kids started changing was remarkable. They were 4th & 5th

68

graders, who some psychologists say aren't yet old enough to be able to make the distinction between their "adult self" and the "child self," but all I can say is baloney! I also had a massage clinic after school on Wednesdays for the kids, and between the two programs the parents couldn't believe what was happening to their children. One child was so timid she rarely talked to her own mother. Her skin, from the neck down, was covered with red sores, she couldn't play in the sun, and her mother had to wrap her in bandages every night because she would bleed all over the sheets. We had only been playing with her inner child's backpack for three weeks, when she rushed in one Monday morning to tell me that she had gone to the mall with her family that weekend and had talked to people. Then when they got home and her Auntie was visiting she had gone up to her and asked her if she would like something to drink. She said, "Mrs. V, my mother is always telling me to go see what Auntie wants to drink when she visits, but I'm too shy. Now I know it's just "Jenny" who is shy, so I say "I love you" and I'm not afraid anymore! By the end of the year she had turned into a chatter box in class and out, could play outside in the sun with no problem, and her skin was 99% clear. Only the very autistic couldn't find their "inner child." Anyway, I didn't mean to make this so long. Thank you for all the wonderful inspiration for all these years.
Suzanne & Suzie Q

There is something very spiritual about tending to your inner child. This transformation of your physical body will be a natural outcome of some very deep and personal inner work. Don't forget, we have no deadline. You have all the time in the world.

Assignment for Chapter Five:

Start a Consumer Report notebook.

Print out four Weekly Progress Reports for a month and start using one.

Make a Wake Up Collar and wear it for 15 minutes before dinner.

Take time for yourself.

Chapter Six:
The Road Trip That Took a Turn

Nelly was really bummed one morning and I woke up with her slumped on my chest waiting for my first conscious, but groggy, moment of awareness to happen.

"What's up little girl?"

"It's not fair! How come everybody else gets to eat goodies and I don't?"

"Oh, you mean the doughnut thing yesterday?"

"Yeah, I'm mad! I wanted one and I didn't get one. Jan got two."

Together we rehashed the reasons behind Nelly's disappointment. It seems the fact that Jan got two doughnuts and was very overweight made Nelly think because she wasn't as big; she should have been able to have *one*. We ended up working out a way to handle all the food situations she didn't think were fair, (a frequent problem in the beginning). I'll tell you all about it in a minute.

Right now, let's go back to the day before for a closer look. We were visiting friends and business associates for four days, and Nelly and I had had 14 weeks of sensible eating under our (smaller) belt. When Terry and I walked into the lobby of their establishment, we were greeted by several acquaintances. Jan, the business owner's daughter smiled at us, and with a doughnut in her hand, she motioned us in.

Nelly wanted one! Her eyes quickly scanned every table and desktop and spied the pink bakery box with the window in the top.

'No,' I said.

She wanted a closer look.

'Okay, but just a look!' While proceeding with the obligatory conversations that separate the civilized from the barbaric, I chatted and preoccupied my way closer to the box, giving very little attention to the business at hand. The lid was closed, but I let Nelly see through the smudged cellophane to the luscious selection of some of her favorite decadences; chocolate-covered glazed doughnuts being her choice for her last supper on death row (if we're ever falsely-accused and convicted). In the course of the morning's events, Nelly insisted on at least six drive-bys of the greasy, pastel carton. She relished several delectable whiffs of the bakery goods inside. Alas, in the end, the ONLY reason we didn't get a doughnut was because no one offered us one and our manners over-rode our desire.

Remembering what happened the day before, I knew Nelly and I needed to have a serious discussion. So I said, "Okay little one, let's talk about this. Tell me how you feel. Get it off your chest."

"It's not fair that Terry can eat three to four times more than we can and not gain an ounce! It's not fair that I don't get to eat what and how much I want anytime I want it! It's not fair! It's not fair! It's not fair!"

"No Nelly it's not fair. In fact life isn't fair, but it's free! We didn't have to pay or do anything to get here and now that we're here, we have to find our own way to be happy with how we are right now. Since we're on the subject, the amount we eat. . ."

"It's not fair."

'No, but guess what?'

"What?"

"Think about something you do get enough of."

"What."

"Well, water for one thing."

"Water? I don't even like water very much."

"That's because you can have all of it you want so it isn't special. If it were special, like in Africa, you would love water and you would think it wasn't fair that somebody got some water and you didn't. You'd think about water all the time the way you think about food now. What else can you think of that you get all you want of?"

"I don't know. Nothin'."

"What about air?"

"What air?"

"See, you get all the air you'll ever need and with every breath you are breathing you don't think one thing about it. Do you know if I held my breath you'd be the first one to rant and rave and turn blue, just to get me to breathe? Talk about fair! You'd be whining and crying until I took in some of this beautiful, free, fresh air."

"Yeah, but air doesn't taste good."

"Well since you brought up the subject, taste is a free gift we've been given, too. If we didn't have a sense of taste, we wouldn't care what we ate. Would you like to give up your sense of taste?"

"No."

"Okay, let's be thankful we can taste and smell. Remember our KISS!"

"Yep! I remember! KISS: Keep It Special, Sweety!"

KISS! Keep It Special Sweety! When we are dealing with food, if we keep the foods that we love 'special' and enjoy them occasionally (I mean occasionally), we'll live a lighter life and we'll be happier.

Once I fully understood where my discontent came from, I was ready to work with Nelly to resolve it and make her happy. I told her how proud I was that she has such good manners and that it saved us from the doughnut. Because I was counting calories at that time, I went to an online calorie counter and typed in doughnut. It was 250 calories, but if I knew then what I know now I would have gone to a carb-counter. A chocolate, glazed doughnut from Dunkin Donuts is 33 grams of carbohydrates. Back then, I asked Nelly, how she would like it if we started keeping track of the calories that we DIDN'T eat so when we turned something down she'd get credit for it.

When I started my new low carb lifestyle, I started keeping track of carbs instead of calories

I bought a small, spiral notebook for Nelly, and now keep track of the carbohydrates she DOESN'T eat. She loves the book and calls it her 'Good Girl' Book.

As you develop a relationship with your little one you'll be able to solve problems that would have remained unconscious. Before I met Nelly I would never have questioned why I was still bummed over not getting a doughnut. Here's an email I want to share from another on-line friend who got to the bottom of an issue because of her close relationship with her inner child.

Dear Pam:
I had a regular screening mammogram come up "abnormal." I was sure there was some mistake, and then the diagnostic mammogram came back "cyst or tumor." The ultrasound said tumor. Next step was biopsy. I lost my appetite during this time, sitting around waiting for the phone to ring with results. I started losing weight a little too fast. I thought, if this is cancer, I will need a lot of energy to get through the treatment. I stopped exercising

and whoa! I went from 130 to 136!

Finally, biopsy day there I was pretending to read magazines in the special waiting room with other terrified women wearing gowns that gaped open in the worst places. Then, half way through the biopsy, the doctor accidently cut into an area she hadn't numbed, and topped it off by hitting a blood vessel.

The cutting hurt like heck, but to stop the bleeding the doctor had to apply heavy pressure right on it. I was in terrible pain when I left.

I was speeding home and there was the Krispy Kreme donut bakery on my side of the road. I was going to have to pass it. A couple traffic lights away, Julianne, my inner child set up a howl. "Let's get a donut! We deserve a donut! We need a treat right now!"

I was agreeing with her, and then I thought no, I just want to get home. That will be treat enough. I can wallow in self-pity there. "But we always get a donut if we're all the way out here!" Julianne insisted. I wavered.

Yes, I thought, we're hardly out this way, and we always do get a donut. "OH LOOK! The 'Hot Now' light is on!" she exclaimed. "Isn't that lucky?!"

Mmmm, the donuts are even better when they've just been pulled out of the hot oil. I decided not to waste this rare opportunity. Donut it was.

We advanced to the next light, and Julianne drooled right over my shoulder. "A hot donut! Maybe two! We could have a glazed, and something with filling and icing! Wonder what today's flavors are?" She was so caught up with it, it was disturbing. Her total engrossment in the flavor snapped me out of it. "No, I'm not stopping after all."

"But we were so good today! We didn't scream when the doctor hit the wrong part even though it really hurt! We just said, 'I can feel that.' And she was so upset when it started bleeding that we had to say it was fine, it didn't hurt, and make a joke so she wouldn't feel bad. That was really HARD! Why do we always have to take care of everyone's feelings and no one takes care of ours? Those donuts are our REWARD."

I kept driving. She was hurling insults. Then a thought popped in my head. "What are you REALLY upset about? What is it you really want?" She stopped long enough to change gears, and the answer was very quiet. "I want to know that everything is going to be OK. I want to know the results will be negative this time."

"And you're going to get that from a *donut*?!!" I asked. Silence. All the way home.

Pam, I think that was the first time I could have had a donut and really wanted to, but I didn't! There were a lot of things I couldn't control about my situation at that point, but I could control what went into my mouth. And within a few days, I was back to 132 pounds.

By the way, Julianne got her wish; the biopsy results came back benign.

Sue

I was so proud of Sue's ability to see the truth behind wanting the doughnut. Often when we just take the time to sit with a craving for a few minutes it passes into the nothingness from whence it came. If it doesn't, that means it's time for some fat; mayonnaise, butter, sour cream, avocado or some other food high in fat.

Sue also shared with me early on, "I tell Julianne she can have anything she wants. . . tomorrow. She seems to be

76

satisfied to wait and invariably she's forgotten about it the next day."

The Bakery Box challenge changed how I handle the 'it's not fair' issue some of us have to deal with.

I've really given this issue of *it's not fair* a lot of deep thought and I think the only way we can come to the conclusion that something is not fair is when we compare ourselves to others. The sooner we stop that, the better. I've written more about the trap of making comparisons in Chapter Nine: *How to Shoot Yourself in the Foot.*

Here is another road trip I'd like to share with you. It came from one of my lovable members of my Make it Fun Club. It almost reads like news from the front lines of a battlefield.

> *I went 200 miles north this week for three days to take care of some business and visit my daughter and best friend.*
>
> *I am so glad Kay (the name for my inner child) and I had started vocalizing. Even better, I've learned to hear her and tell her, "NO."*
>
> *I ate what I believed to be a filling breakfast before leaving the house for my road trip. My inner child and my 12-year-old son ganged up on me and tried REALLY hard to convince me that we were starved and should stop and eat.*
>
> *"McDonald's coming up!"*
>
> *"We've only been on the road an hour; it's only been a few hours since we had breakfast."*
>
> *"But it's McDonald's and WE ARE STARVING!"*
>
> *"No we are not, this is habit hunger. Road trip = eating."*

"Hey! SUBWAY ."

"No."

"DAN'S FAMILY RESTAURANT."

"No."

"CRACKER BARREL."

"No."

"BUT WE LOVE CRACKER BARREL!"

"No."

"BUT WE ALWAYS EAT AT A CRACKER BARREL ON A ROAD TRIP AND I AM HUNGRY!"

"No."

Oh, it wasn't easy. I finally made a deal with myself, my inner child, and my child.

"We will eat when we get to Joliet. It will be four hours since we had breakfast by the time we get food in Joliet."

"BUT THERE'S FOOD NOW"

"There's no White Castle. We are having White Castle."

Okay so it wasn't the best thing to pick but it was the only place to eat where there were none of them until we hit Joliet. It worked! We made it to White Castle without too much whining from either of the two children.

-Karen and Kay.

Karen has learned that travel is tricky and the fast food business has figured out they have a real influence on our travelling minds. Those 60 foot road signs beckoning you to Burger King aren't cheap. They know us better than we know ourselves. . . until we wake-up and realize what's going on.

If Karen would have packed some vegetable snacks and a cooler with hard boiled eggs and slices of turkey, beef or chicken and some mayonnaise for the trip, her "kids" would not have even noticed the signs and the habit of travel-hunger would have been doused with good food.

Don't let your next road trip or party cause you to take a turn. In chapter seven I'll tell you my experiences eating out in restaurants and give you some ideas for staying on your program which will also help you with road trips and parties.

Assignment for Chapter Six:

Print out four Weekly Progress Reports for a month. Start today (even if it's not Monday) and begin using the report! You will be hooked once you do.

Start a Good Girl Notebook and become aware of the foods high in carbs that you pass up so you can give your inner child her credit due.

Look for ways you are beginning to see with new eyes.

Chapter Seven:
Look Out!

Earlier, I told you about a spat I had with Nelly. Her Consumer Report came out of that spat. I hope you've started one for your own inner child. Let's take a closer look at what happened that day:

The day had started to turn on me that morning when I got back from my walk dripping in sweat with my husband informing me that the air conditioning wasn't working. (I found out I'm not as nice as I thought I was). As the day wore on and the temperature outside hit 112 degrees, I told him I wouldn't be cooking in our 95-degree kitchen; we'd be eating out. The second Nelly heard the words, 'eating out,' she began to plot. This was a Wednesday, and I knew we had a banquet to go to on Saturday. So I knew that if I gave-in to Nelly this day, I'd give in on Saturday. (You know what you know.) Instead of putting a gentle foot down, I allowed her to "work" me throughout the afternoon. It escalated into a nasty, name-calling brawl. If we'd been married, I would have been on the phone to the divorce lawyer.

Because I'd been playing with Nelly for so long this was testimony to the fact that this relationship was alive with emotion. And even though generally we have a wonderful time together, I was reminded that occasionally I would be spending a night on the couch.

In the end, we stayed home. I cooked and Nelly sulked the entire evening. The next morning, after a great night's sleep, I was able to see the event more clearly and glean some much needed wisdom from the experience. It was then that I realized how important it is to keep track of everything we eat, not just what we don't eat

The experience made me see with new eyes that if we have allowed ourselves to become overweight, we have allowed ourselves too many carbs. For instance, if we don't know the carb count on a food we could easily knock back 100 without a thought

Obesity is surging in the U.S. and the researchers are going nuts trying to figure out what to do with us. A recent survey (2010) was conducted by Consumer Report which found four out of ten Americans admitted being "somewhat overweight" and 11% said they were very overweight or obese. The researchers at the Centers for Disease Control and Prevention say that 68% of Americans are overweight or obese. That means there's a whole lot of denial goin' on kiddies.

I read an article in My Health News and Molly Kimball, a registered dietitian at Ochshner's Elmwood Fitness Center in New Orleans said, "There does seem to be a disconnect between reality and the answers most of us give when asked questions about our diet. So many people think that what they're eating is healthy — diet frozen dinners, fat-free ice cream, 100-calorie pretzel packs. Or they say, 'I never eat fast food,' but that doesn't mean they're not eating a lot of other unhealthy things. Part of the disconnect comes from the way foods are marketed to us." Molly's right on.

I love to imagine what goes on in marketing and advertising meetings like in the movie *What Women Want*. I picture a big conference table with about twenty creative advertisers and marketers together to discuss packaging and marketing like what Molly talked about. Remember these people do NOT market to the adult; they go straight to the kid in us. Here's what I imagine Walter, the head of advertising, would say addressing his team for the up-coming campaign for a product.

"Okay folks....let's quiet down.....let's quiet down

"Here is our challenge.....We just finished 2010 and our sales are not what they should be. So I told the research department to get out there and get me some answers and here's what their tellin' me now.

"They're tellin' me people are anxious about eatin' healthy these days. They're lookin' for words like healthy, nutritious, fiber-filled, fat-free and what not. So we gotta put a lot of those words on the *front* of our packages from now on. We gotta increase those sales.

"The law says we have to put the ingredients on the package...we know that... but thanks to our lobbyists we can put those on the back and we can make the print so small it'll be hard to read! Whatever we pay the lobbyists was sure worth it for those two things.

"Where's Rita...Rita raise your hand...ok..Rita over there, the law says we have to put the sugar content on the package, but it does not say we have to put it in ounces so were gonna put it in grams. Nobody knows what a gram is so they'll go blank on that one and never know how much sugar really is in it. And here's what the legal department told me...... they say we can list part of the sugar as fructose....those dumbos out there don't know that fructose really is sugar too. In fact we can call it high fructose...makes it sound really good for you that way.

"Bill, did a *KILLER* job on this photo ! It takes me right back to my mama's home cookin! Great job Bill! The best part is you made the portion size H-U-G-E. Hey, people don't have a clue what a portion is.

"Harley suggested we tell 'em those big portions ARE "diet" size. What IS diet size anyway? *They* sure don't know. Or better yet let's think up words that don't really tell the size, like, uh, Wise Size or Perfect Size. Jennifer came up with this one...Size Six Size. That's a good one considering how much sugar and high fructose we put it there.

"Now listen to this 'cause the key is we need folks to *believe* they're eatin' healthy even if they aren't. It isn't our fault that they eat too much and too much sugar and too much high fructose and wind up gettin' fat. They gotta be responsible for themselves. All we care about is they eat the big portions so they'll have to buy more...faster. We gotta make sure the CEO gets his big bonus each year.

"So come on folks let's get to work on this right now."

The way I see it, you (really your inner child) is up against a multi-billion dollar industry that has some of the brightest and cleverest minds putting their heads together to get your little one's attention. Until you get a firm hold on your inner child, when you go to the grocery store you're like a child with free reign at a candy shop or toy store.

One thing that has really helped me is what I call the "parking lot" talk. I used it a great deal when I was climbing out of debt. It goes something like this:

"Okay, Nelly, we're going into the grocery store and we've got our list and I don't want you to give me any trouble. I know there will be temptations, but if we stay on the outside parts of the store and only go in the inner aisles to get mustard and mayonnaise, we'll be fine. However, if you give me any trouble, we'll leave and you won't get anything."

In the beginning, I found I had to be very careful at the checkout counter. Once while loading groceries into my trunk I noticed a sack of Hershey Kisses in the top of one of my bags. I realized it was a last-minute purchase at checkout. The candy is put there (by those wise marketers) to get the kids to want it while waiting in line.

I vaguely remembered adding the candy to my purchases (that's how tricky Nelly is). Once I "woke up" I marched that bag of candy (and Nelly) back in the store and got a refund. I told the man I bought the candy on accident. When you undue a mistake like that your inner child will be impressed. Nelly has NEVER messed with the checkout candy since.

Molly (from the article I mentioned) also said, "Skip the front of the package, and turn it over to read the ingredients." What she failed to say was, don't even look at the calorie count, just look at the carbohydrate count. My friend Leanne Ely, the author of Saving Dinner tells us if, when you read the ingredients on a label you can't pronounce even one of them put the package back! Have you ever noticed some stuff on the shelves of our grocery stores have hundreds of ingredients and most are unpronounceable?

I have a challenge for you. Stop reading labels. If you buy a chicken there is no list of ingredients; it's just that, a chicken. It's the same with , cabbage, broccoli, eggplant, eggs, tomatoes and such. See how much unprocessed food you can cut out of your diet in the next year by buying fresh unprocessed food. (All the fresh stuff is around the outside of a grocery store. The processed stuff is in the middle aisles.)

Deborah Enos said in that same article, "Sugar is the number one health challenge we're fighting in this country. People have no idea what's an appropriate amount. And because sugar is the only element of food for which there's no *daily recommended* amount given on the back of food labels, most people don't know how much is too much. Any sugar is too much. Remember what I said about why we have a sweet tooth. It's normal to want sweet food, but now we are grown up and we don't need mother's milk any longer, but we still need the love. If every time you crave something sweet you took a time-out for some one-on-one attention to your inner child following the five steps I outlined in chapter three, your cravings soon disappear.

Years ago, one of my Weight Watcher leaders told me I had a fat mind! To illicit that response I'd said, "If I go off program in a particular hour by eating a cookie (we were to keep a log of every hour of our waking day telling whether we stayed on or fell off the program) and have to put an X in that hour's square, I may as well go off the program for the whole hour and eat a bunch of cookies!"

She was right. I did have a fat mind. I completely missed the reason we were tracking. I was more concerned with getting an X in a square than the amount of calories I was consuming. Can you guess the age of that fat little mind?

One day, while printing out another Weekly Progress Report, I realized that by tracking my thoughts along with Nelly's Consumer Report and her Good Girl Report, Nelly was getting attention. When I sit down to write the good and the bad, she's right there. Often I'll write the whole report for the day, the morning after, since the day before is still fresh in my mind. Even though we had piddledinked around for 11 of the first 16 weeks we were on the program, vacillating about five pounds, the fact that I had kept track kept me from quitting. I think tracking keeps you alert. If you quit tracking before you have turned into a thin person thinker about food, you'll go right back into being a fat person thinker about it.

Whenever Nelly sees her three-ring binder with her reports in it, she smiles. It's like being back in school again when Mrs. Brose, my fourth grade teacher, tracked everything I did. This made me feel special. Remember, this project is more about awareness, patience, joy, creativity, appreciation, persistence and love than it is about weight-loss. As you track your little one, you are loving her and giving her attention, and she will blossom in the light you shine on her.

I'd like to discuss another issue here, and that's portion control. When you eat a high carbohydrate diet you need to abide by portion control, but when on a high fat, restricted carbohydrate diet, portion control isn't very necessary. For an example: In the first eight months of my new lifestyle I went through what I called my "Clinton Phase." Remember when our president was asked why he did what he did to Monica Lewinsky? Remember his answer? "Because I could." In my Clinton Phase I was eating approximately 4,000 calories a day! Most of the calories were from fat and hardly any from carbohydrates because I'd limited mine to 10 to 15 grams a day which would be around 200 calories because the carbohydrate foods were vegetables. The bottom line, I lost five pounds in those eight months! Now I'm over my Clinton Phase and I probably consume about 2,800 calories today (I'm not sure because I don't count them anymore). What you will discover for yourself is that when you are on a restricted carbohydrate diet you don't store fat when you eat it.

It's the fat that stops any form of craving. In fact early in my transition when I'd crave a dessert or a starch, if I would immediately go to the refrigerator and eat a tablespoon of mayonnaise and a couple branches of broccoli, the craving would disappear within 30 seconds. It was just like magic. I found out that there is something in your brain that's triggered by the intake of fat that automatically shuts down cravings. What a miracle body we have.

One day in September, I was feeling sorry for myself and I knew Nelly was behind it. So I got a glass of ice water and I sat in my favorite chair and asked like I always do, "What's up little one."

"It's that dumb magazine!"

We'd gotten the October Better Homes & Gardens magazine that morning in the mail and on the cover were beautiful sugar cookies cut in fall leaf shapes and covered in sprinkles of sugar. I remember thinking, 'I don't bake cookies anymore,' but I was in the middle of a project and brushed off the thought. Nelly didn't, hence the sad feeling. So we talked about it.

"I know it's very sad we can't have sugar anymore and it cuts out all the fun we had with the grandkids rolling out the dough, cutting out the cookies and decorating them. It's over so we're going to have to replace that with something else. Do you have any ideas?"

"No. I don't like it one bit! Everybody gets to have sugar cookies in the fall and Christmas is coming and what about those cookies?"

"We can't start eating sugar just because it's Christmas Nelly. Again we have to come up with alternatives."

"Again, we have to come up with alternatives! I hate that."

"Listen Nell, you don't have to get sassy, no mocking please. I can't have you getting all upset just because a magazine comes in the mail. Just wait until Christmas comes and the stores are full of Christmas treats and then there'll be Easter, and birthdays and every damn holiday is going to be immersed in sugar."

"It's not fair! It's not fair! What are we gonna do?"

"We are going to think of alternatives and you are going to come up with some fun things. For starters I have an idea for what we can do with the sack of flour we still haven't tossed. You know how we decided it wasn't fair to give it to the poor people, because it's not good for any of us humans to eat no matter what our socio-economic profile is."

"Socio-economic profile? That's a hard word. So what's your idea?"

"Well, you know how kids have so many stuffed animals and there are two huge shelves of them at the Goodwill?"

"Yeah.'

"I've always thought of stuffed animals as an American natural resource. They seem to reproduce on their own there is such a glut of them."

"Yeah, so you want to give the flour to them?"

"No, silly, I want to use them for bases for lamps and book ends in kids' bedrooms."

"Huh?"

"First I'd pick an animal the size I want and I'd perform a minor surgery on the tummy, take out some of the stuffing and replace the void with a heavy, smooth river rock and stitch it back up. Then, and here's where the flour comes in, I'd paper Mache the whole toy. Then I'd paint it using acrylic paint and put a clear plastic paint over the finished paint and voila, I'll use up the flour and create a great gift for a child's bedroom!"

"I want one, I want one! I can't wait to make some. Can we make one today? Huh, can we, can we?"

"Yes, if you'll get yourself out of the funk you've been in. You've been weighing on me."

"Okay, I'm happy. Let's play."

Assignment for Chapter Seven:

The next time you go grocery shopping; have a parking lot talk in your car before you go in. Remember it's you and your little one against the big world of hype. Take a list and stay away from the center of the store as much as you can.

Keep tracking.

Continue to keep an open dialogue with your inner child. Get to the bottom of problems as they arise.

Chapter Eight

Let's Eat Out!

In the past when you were losing weight, eating in restaurants no doubt presented problems for you. This is because the moment you sit down, you go into "entitlement" mode. You are there to be served and it feels so good! You go from always being the server to being THE SERVED. You are queen for an hour or so! It just doesn't get any better than that. You are royalty, and your inner child is in her element. Go ahead and bask in that element, but don't forget the five pounds you're working on. Go ahead and enjoy the wonderful aroma of the food being cooked and take pleasure when the server brings your food and says, "Enjoy."

The tricky part is that a restaurant is the perfect place for your inner child to act up if she's going to. It's the same as when your birth kids know you are distracted on the phone, they'll tend to get rowdy. You need to be prepared. Here are some strategies that will help.

1. Have a "parking lot" talk with your inner child before you go in the restaurant. It can go something like this: 'Okay little one, remember what we *really* want.' (State your inner child's reason for going along with your new lifestyle. You both agree that you're not going to carry around that extra weight anymore. Also, use all the ammo you have if your class reunion is in three weeks, bathing suit weather is just around the corner, you want your neighbor to think you're cute, or whatever.) Since Nelly was so appalled by the fact that she was lugging around seven sacks of flour, my parking lot talks went something like this: 'Just think, Nell, we have dumped four sacks and only have three sacks left to lose and then we will look even better than we do now! You are

doing so well and I'm very proud of you! I love you.'

2. Take your five-pound brick or whatever you've chosen to use with you in a tote bag. Lugging it in the restaurant will keep you focused on your resolve. Either set it on the table or keep it in your lap.

3. See if you can down a glass of water while you wait for your food.

4. If you are dining with someone, take advantage of the conversation to distract your inner child from what the other people get to have.

5. When your meal is served, this is the perfect time to have one more talk with your sweet little child before you dig in. Just close your eyes and say a few words to her. The beauty of this talk is, you won't get "put away" for talking to yourself in public, because fellow diners will just think you're on Blue Tooth or saying grace. (You could actually say grace while you're at it.) 'Okay, Nelly, you've been so good at practicing turning a bite into the consistency of baby food that you don't ever have to count chews anymore! And I'm so proud of you for telling the waiter not to bring the bread. And ordering "the works" for the baked potato, but not the potato was fun, wasn't it! We can put all of it on your steak. Doesn't it look and smell so good? I love you!'

6. Ask the server for a "doggy bag" as soon as your meal is served. Restaurants are notorious for serving too much food to us, so transfer the excess to the container before you start eating. Oh and here's a novel idea! Really give the contents of the doggy bag to your dog when you get home.

7. When the chance for dessert comes . . . pass if it's not a special, special occasion. If the restaurant wheels out a dessert cart you can do what Suzanne told me she does. (Suzanne is the one you heard

91

about earlier who wrote to me about the make believe backpacks.)

She writes:

Dear Pam,

When my inner kiddy wants junk food, and we go into battle, I can stop the battle with the first shot. Whenever I went to my favorite grocery store, my little princess always went wild when we'd have to go past the incredible 35- foot-long bakery counter. The smells were (are) so heavenly, and I often gave in when she begged for a doughnut. One day I thought to tell her she could have anything she wanted, but I was going to pass. She got to go wild selecting whatever she wanted, but it was pretend. The only stipulation was that she couldn't put the results on my body. It's so odd, but my craving went away, while my little inner child chowed down on all her favorite things, and I found that I could enjoy watching her take such pleasure in whatever it was she wanted, without it affecting my waistline. It's much cheaper that way too! Now I pack a bag for her each morning. Sometimes she likes a fancy bag, sometimes a backpack, and we put in things that she likes to play with as well as things she might like to eat that day. She must have a freezer in there, because ice cream seems to go in occasionally, along with peanut butter sandwiches and marshmallows and Big Hunks. These bags are kind of like the tent in the Harry Potter movie because sometimes we pack in a pony or maybe a swimming pool. Toys and games I haven't thought of since childhood often end up in there too. In the evening when I'm going to bed, I spend a second or two to empty the bag and thank her for helping me all day. Tomorrow I'll check to see what color her backpack will be and what will go in it. It's much more fun loving her than fighting her.
Suzanne in California

Suzanne has discovered the key to this whole new way to lose weight! The more we can practice using our imaginations, the more fun we can have with this. Think about this; there is more to enjoy about going to a restaurant than the food. Here are some of the non-food pleasures I came up with. See if you can come up with more.

1. I don't have to cook.
2. I get to be waited on.
3. I don't have to wash dishes and scour pots and pans.
4. I get to experience a different atmosphere.
5. It is a special occasion.
6. I don't have a begging dog at my feet.
7. I get to dress up and go out.
8. I might see some of my friends.
9. I get to have matching plates, silverware and glasses.

One more thing while I'm on the subject of restaurants:

I have made a rule that when ordering dinner in a restaurant I usually order seafood. I know fish is a very healthy entre choice but I don't enjoy cooking it and I'd rather let the restaurant smell like fish instead of my kitchen.

Today I look forward to going to a restaurant as a very special occasion where food is the side effect. My food is not the center of my life, but an interesting necessity, like a fancy handle on the toilet.

Assignment for Chapter Eight:

Start a fresh Weekly Progress Report

Get a tote bag to hold your five pound weight and take it with you into the restaurant.

See if you can come up with some other pleasures that go with dining out.

Chapter Nine:
How to Shoot Yourself in the Foot

Shooting yourself in the foot can be an accident when you play with a gun and don't know how it works. It can also be on purpose when for some *crazy* reason you deem it a valid action.

You certainly didn't collect your weight on purpose. We shoot ourselves in the foot every time we don't stop to figure out how *we* work. That takes time. It takes time on a daily basis to understand what makes you tick.

"Know thyself," the philosopher tells us.

When I was in denial about my weight, one of the biggest forces keeping me struggling was my penchant for judging others and comparing myself to them. For five years I sang in a Sweet Adeline Chorus made up of 130 women whose average age was 55 and average weight I'd guess was 175 pounds. I've never in my life seen such a massive collection of overweight, middle-aged women. When I compared my body to the average singer in that group I felt – *little*.

But I was shooting myself in the foot. That tendency to compare cost me five years of dragging around seven sacks of flour. I look back and wonder how I could have considered myself *little*. Had I been minding my own business I would not have judged any of those women. They have nothing to do with me and my weight problem. But I allowed comparing myself to them make me feel better about myself. Is there nine-year-old mentality lurking around here?

I haven't been singing with the chorus for several years now and rarely see any of those women any more. Now I understand that the overweight women in that group had no more to do with me *then* than they do *now.* It's ridiculous to hide our problems behind someone with bigger problems. I had to stop feeling better about myself in comparison to those who had more to lose than I did.

This fallacy can work the other way, too. You can look at someone who has a beautiful, healthy body and think, 'I'll never have that,' or 'It's not fair.' Both comparisons are an exact example of shooting yourself in the foot.

When we stop looking outside ourselves to feel good or bad and just focus on what we really want (a happy, healthy body that is easy to play in) we are on the right track. Just keep remembering this: Your reason to keep going is you don't want to carry the weight anymore. Whether or not you change is dependent on the types of food you eat and the activities you take part in. But the food and activities depend on you remembering what you really want.

While outlining the writing of this book I recalled a woman whom I'd known for the five years I was in the chorus. She weighed 125 pounds and was five feet, seven inches tall. We talked on one occasion about weight. She said she once weighed 185 pounds. Since I'd never seen her heavy I was shocked to hear that. I decided to give her a call and ask her some questions about how she lost the weight. What made her decide to lose? How had she kept the weight off?

Her name is Ruth Peterson and here's what she had to say.

"The decision to lose the weight took a few weeks to digest into my mind and heart. My brother-in-law had an almost fatal heart attack and he weighed the same as I did, 185 pounds. I remember thinking first, 'I'm glad it's not me.' Then I wished a doctor would tell me I'd have a fatal heart attack if I didn't lose this weight! How dumb was that? Well, as soon as that thought was out, it hit me: Why do I need a doctor to tell me I'll die, if I don't do something? But then it took me a few weeks of watching my bother-in-law start losing weight, getting fit and feeling better and better before I got serious about the whole thing. It didn't happen overnight. The other issues I had and still have are Fibromyalgia and weak knees. My knees were killing me. I thought that if I didn't do something my knees were going to get worse. I worried that I would get fatter and I didn't want to live that way anymore."

I asked her how long it took her to lose the 60 pounds (12 sacks of flour) and she said it took a whole year, but she'd heard the faster you lose weight the faster you'll gain it back. When I asked her how long she has weighed 125 she really had to think. She was shocked when she backed up through the years to remember when the whole process started and she was amazed to tell me she'd weighed 125 pounds for ten years! I asked her if she could ever go back to her old thinking that caused the 185 pounds and she said unequivocally, "NO!"

We talked for more than an hour. Here are a few other points from that conversation that I thought were very interesting. She said, "I put up a photo of myself in a blouse that was bursting at the buttons. I hated the photo and it made me hate me! Every time I saw it I got mad and after a while I realized I was going at this all wrong. I needed to get to the point where I liked me right where I was.

I needed to feel good about myself right then, because I knew I was going to get this weight off, no doubt in my mind. So I went out and bought a small wardrobe of clothes that fit. I looked nice and I felt happy in the clothes. (They were 1X.) It was a real turning point because the nice clothes changed my self-image and allowed me to be what I was; a large woman who looked good. That wardrobe kept me on the diet and that's when I really started losing the weight. In a very short time I gave those clothes away (and they were almost like brand new!). Then I went into a size smaller and did the same thing. For me it was very important that I felt good about myself while I was making this drastic change."

This tactic helped Ruth because her motive to change was a health issue. She had her brother-in-law as her sack of flour if you will. Ruth felt good about herself at each turn along the way and has ended up wearing a size 6 for the past ten years! She told me she really watches what she eats. If she eats too rich a food or too much, she gets sick to her stomach.

I asked her about snacking. She looked around her kitchen and said, "When I think of a snack I think of fruit like apples, a plum or berries or vegetables. I've always felt God didn't create junk (as in junk food) and fruits and vegetables are as close to what God created for us as anything we put into our mouths. I also don't deprive myself of anything I really want. But I only take a little bit. I've learned that I don't need much. There is also the 90/10 rule. If you are eating healthy 90% of the time, 10% of not so healthy eating is just fine if it keeps you from feeling deprived."

Without telling Ruth about Nelly I asked her if through the whole process she had come to learn more about herself. She answered, "Oh yes! I look back and I am so thankful that I had the challenge because it brought me to a better understanding of me and an appreciation of who I am. I am God's child. I learned that I have a wonderful imagination that serves me well. I am able to look at a Toll House Chocolate Chip Cookie and see Crisco and imagine eating a teaspoon of that instead of the cookie. I can look at French fries or potato chips and in my mind's eye put them on a napkin and see the grease ooze out of them onto the napkin.

I didn't know Ruth when she had 12 sacks of flour to lose so I don't know how the loss of them changed her, but I know it had to have made a difference in her self-esteem. She is so comfortable in her body and has a poise that reflects an inner power. She made up her mind to change and she did change.

From now on, only compare you to you.

Another way we shoot ourselves in the foot is by unconscious eating. Every bite we take that is unconscious is a habit bite. The habit bites we take in a day directly affect our weight. A habit bite is a bite we often don't even remember taking. A habit bite is void of emotion and therefore taste.

Do you know what taste has as a constant companion? Emotion. There is something so wonderful about that first bite when all your awareness is focused on the morsel of food and the taste.

By the tenth bite, emotion has left the room. Whenever habitual and routine eating occurs emotion disappears. Much of my eating was robotical. I discovered when I stay alert to the bite about to go into my mouth I enjoy it. Every bite taken unconsciously is joyless.

Here is a poem I wrote about unconscious eating.

I Can't Believe I Ate it!

I made myself a sandwich but something's really weird
The crumbs are on the counter, but the sandwich . . .
disappeared
I can't believe I ate it and I won't admit I did
I know I took a bite or two while I was screwing on the lid
To the gallon jar of mayonnaise, after licking off the knife
That was standing knee deep in there, treading mayonnaise for
its life
I might have eaten just a half of that sandwich that I made

I know I washed some down with a glass of lemonade
That I drank to quench my awful thirst after eating guacamole
Or maybe it was taco chips, or NO the crescent roll see
I smeared some peanut butter on the roll and took a taste
When my buds relayed the message that unless I heaped in
haste
A glob of homemade jelly on the butter and the roll
The overall experience would leave a gourmet hole
So I carried out the order, drank some milk to wash it down
And when I took the carton back, you won't believe it but I
found
A Snickers bar I'd started and didn't have time to finish
So I'd hidden it with forethought in a box of frozen spinach
Which I bought for just that reason 'cause the kids are little
snackers
I've learned from past experience they'll eat you out of crackers
And anything that's salty and everything that's sweet
They're worse than ants at picnics when it comes to finding
treats
Which brings me back to wonder if that's what happened to my
sandwich
Did the children spy my meal and fail to understand which
Food is theirs and this is mine? It's hard to keep things
separate
Those sneaky little snackers must have gotten awfully
desperate
Okay, if I did consume it and I must admit I'm stuffed
Then where's that little voice I have that says I've had enough?
I remember reading about Mr. Hunger Pang
It said he lives ten minutes even if his hungry fang
Hasn't bitten into something that he tells me that I crave
I like the thought that I can make a hunger pang behave
I guess it's pretty obvious by looking at my hips
That more than meats and vegetables have passed between my
lips

A small bite here, a swallow there, just how much I can't
remember
But according to my scale, I've gained ten pounds since last
September

No, we don't shoot ourselves in the foot on purpose. We do it unconsciously. That's why it's so important to wake up and taste every morsel as if it is our first bite. Tasting every bite slows down eating which gives your inner child time to tell you she is getting full.

Someone once said, "Hunger is the best sauce." I've played with that notion as I documented my last three years slow poking my way to my goal. I have found that I enjoy being hungry because it makes my meal taste better when it's time to eat. A snack robs me of the sauce produced by hunger! As the hour approaches for a meal, instead of eating a snack, I let my hunger come into play for the sole purpose of enjoying it. One low carb doctor told me he rates his hunger on a scale of one to ten and he tries to let it get to a six before he has a meal. In order to play with this, you have to intend to enjoy the feeling of being hungry. By playing my hunger game I have learned the difference between real hunger and false hunger brought on by habit. Nelly and I have talked a lot about habit hunger in this book; that it's what you experience after you've eaten dinner and you're watching TV and you think, 'popcorn sounds good,' or 'I wonder if there's any ice cream left?' You're really not hungry; you just want to eat while you watch the program.

If you want to play with your hunger, try this: skip lunch and don't snack in the afternoon. You will start really becoming hungry around 2:00 pm and your inner child will start messing with you. You'll be minding your own business and you'll find yourself in the kitchen without remembering you walked in there. If you are at work, you'll catch yourself diving into your purse for money for the snack machine. Your sense of smell will be acute and you'll smell people's gum, and if you take a walk in the area of restaurants you'll become like a hunting dog ruled by your nose. If you want to try this be sure to be in full control of your portions at dinner and remember to eat mindfully or you could turn this learning experience into an over-eating session!

I'm not telling you not to snack; I think sensible snacks keep our systems running optimally. I'm just suggesting understanding what real hunger feels like, because most of us don't. Just think, in our caveman days we were hungry a lot! Our main concern was on survival, so we didn't have time to think about much else. I'll bet most of our prayers back then were for food for survival. Today, we have an abundance of food and now we pray for help to lose weight. We are so fortunate!

By keeping a close and loving relationship going with your inner child you will be more alert and awake when it's time to eat. You'll be able to talk to your Nelly when she starts to compare or judge. Ultimately you will change your eating life. You'll be able to look back and say, "I can't believe I ever weighed that," and as Ruth said, "Oh yes! I look back and I am so thankful that I had the weight challenge because it brought me to a better understanding of me and an appreciation of who I am. I am God's child." My prayer is you make it your first priority to get to know your inner child on this weight dumping journey and that the absence of all that extra weight becomes automatic result of you getting to know and love who you are. You are God's child.

Assignment for Chapter Nine:

Keep tracking your inner child with the Weekly Progress Report.

Make a list of the ways you shoot yourself in the foot.

Stop Comparing.

Feel good in your clothing knowing the size you buy is temporary.

Chapter Ten:
Think Adorable

Terry and I go to an annual charity banquet on Deer Island on the Columbia River. Deer Island is a working cattle ranch and breeding facility for thoroughbred race horses. I love to go there every year because I adore horses, farms, barns and hay, and we get to dress in black tie and blue jeans! I always wear a sparkly top, jeans and cowboy boots that only get to come out and play one day a year.

Terry is the emcee of the event because he was in television for 20 years in his past, and I love seeing him in a tux on top and jeans on the bottom. The other thing I love about the perennial party is the food. Dave, the owner of the island ranch, barbeques a whole hind quarter (or two) for the shindig. The rest of the food is catered by a fabulous restaurant in Portland.

Back when I was in a new mindset about my weight, I went to the party in 'learning mode.' Food was not going to be my dominant reason to go! At the party, I was seated next to a thin woman named Velma and her husband, Bill. They were in their seventies. I asked the woman if this was her first time at the gala, and she said, "Oh, no, we've come for three years."

Because she was in such great shape for her age, I asked her, "What is the main reason you come here for this fundraiser?"

She said, "I love this ranch and I love to see the people I know and meet new people." That's when the conversation thickened.

"So, is that how you look at all parties you go to?"

"What d'you mean?"

"Do you ever think of food first? Like, 'oh the church potluck is tonight I wonder what good food will be there?'"

"Oh, no I don't think I think about the food ever. But I do go to church and we do have potlucks."

"So when you get an invitation to a party, what IS the first thing you think of?"

At this point Bill chimed in and said, "How to get out of it."

We laughed and then she said, "I think about seeing the people and having fun talking to them and hearing what they are up to since the last time I saw them."

After that discussion, I decided to conduct a little investigation. I saw a woman a couple tables away from us I know who is thin, tan, and lovely. (That night she wore a black leather halter top.) We hugged and I said after the customary blah, blah blahs, "When you were getting ready to come to this party, did you think about food?" She laughed and said, "NO" the way you'd answer if you'd been asked the stupidest question in the world. Like, 'Do you like to eat raw slugs?'

After dinner the desserts started coming out! They were glorious! Velma watched as a woman in a white chef uniform complete with the hat walked past our table with a scrumptious blueberry cheesecake. She said, "Oh I wish I wanted some of that. It looks delicious."

Those were words from a thin mind. I made a note on my Weekly Progress Report that very soon I would be able to think that way automatically. "Oh I wish I wanted some of that. It looks delicious," instead of "I'm stuffed, but I've gotta have some of that."

I think this is a good place to tell you that as you become less preoccupied with food and more aware of your "thinking" you'll begin to listen to the "quiet voice" and you'll have food left on your plate. This is the time to say to yourself, "I wish I still wanted this." And instead of saying, "(sniff) goodbye, I have to throw you out," say, "I'm going to put you in a little container and have you later as a snack."

Early on my journey to a lighter life I sent an email out to all my subscribers asking those who were *thin* to respond in one sentence telling me how they regard food. It was enlightening. As you read their comments pause and let those thoughts you'd like to be part of your thinking, sink in. Reread out loud those that resonate with you.

Before I read their thoughts, consider thinking healthy rather than thin. I specifically asked these respondents to reply if they were thin. Nelly was the one who wanted to be thin and together we had to change the adjective to healthy. We have to be careful of the term thin. I don't want to ever feel "boney." I've hugged thin people and thought 'Oh, too thin.' I don't want to be a boney hugger. In time I changed the adjective to adorable. In other words, you need to know what you want to look like, not weigh.

To find out what I wanted to look like, half way through my journey I started body shopping. My stepdaughter, Kristi Marsh, has the most beautiful body and I wanted mine to look like hers, but she's taller and younger than I am, so I had re-think that one. When I'd be out and about and see a body I thought looked great, I'd check out the length and age of it too. One day I was at a spiritual retreat and while washing my hands in the women's restroom on a break, I noticed this darling woman next to me. She was about my age, my height and had the same size frame, so I said, "Excuse me, you have a beautiful body. I want one just like it. So, how much does it weigh?" (I know you can't just go up to people and ask something like that unless you know the person would take it the right way.

I had my wedding rings on so I knew she knew I wasn't hitting on her. Besides, almost everyone at this retreat would know we are not our bodies. We are way more than the physical part we use and can see.) She laughed and even hugged me because she took my comments and question as a compliment, which of course they were. Then she said, "Thank you! It weighs 135 pounds." Wow, there before me was the body I wanted and the weight I wanted to be. Not 120 like I weighed in high school when I taught ballet and worked out with the rally squad almost every day. Just a perfect weight for a woman on Social Security, who loves life, exercises reasonably, doesn't want to drag around seven sacks of flour and wants to look ADORABLE.

I weigh 135 pounds and it's just right for me! You can start looking for the look you want and it will encourage your inner child to cooperate all the more. Be careful when deciding on a new body that you aren't influenced by Hollywood. We're constantly given unattainable images from models on the covers of magazines to actresses in the movies and on television. Many of you played with Barbie Dolls and know her body shape is not real and completely unattainable unless you had surgery to remove your lower ribs. Put all that fantasy behind you and find a body that's the same height and age as yours and one you can adore.

Make sure when you body shop you do it just to find the body you like and don't be comparing yourself *now* to your future body. I think you can only shoot yourself in the foot by comparing if it causes you to deny your own problem. Just use the body you find to your liking as your goal body. And remember weighing what that goal body weighs is not as important as getting to know and love <u>you</u> more.

Now that I have the "thin" thing out of the way, here's what "the thin" had to say:

My thoughts on food: Food is fuel for your body; if you overfill your tank, you'll have a mess. If you use the wrong type of fuel, it may not run right.
~ *Heather*

People assumed I was living a virtuous life of self-denial. It wasn't true! I had a thyroid disorder and could no more help being thin than a large person with a medical disorder can help being large. But I was perceived as somehow *better*. There is no virtue in self-denial of that sort. What a bunch of hooey! When people found out that it was a medical issue, they considered me lucky. Strange, because untreated, it often leads to depression and can lead to heart trouble.

My cat nearly died of the same thing. With her, people recognized that she was ill. I have been told all my life I was thin. I am not really anymore, I am small framed and close to my healthiest weight. However, my image of myself is still thin, and even more interesting, people still think of me as thin.
~ *Elizabeth*
PS: I did get the thyroid disorder under control and feel MUCH better, and so does the cat.

If you really want to know how thin people think about food, I know from hanging around them! They don't THINK about food ever. They eat because they have to or their children are begging for food. They wait until they are shaky and then they eat. It doesn't consume their life. Unlike my father who is not thin and THINKS about food all the time. If we are going somewhere at one, he has us go early to get something to eat. So I guess in theory, it comes right down to whether you THINK about food or not.

~ Stacy

Being thin is as much a problem for us "thin people" as it is for "fat people." Most of us want to be just an average size so it won't be so difficult in finding clothes and shoes to wear. Also, all the comments said in envy, such as "Wish I could give you some of my fat!" or "Be careful--a puff of wind might come along and blow you away!" hurt our feelings.

~ Dee

I weigh 112 on a "fat" day. I think of healthy food as the best medicine; it keeps me happy and energized. I think of unhealthy food as poison: it makes me sleepy and sick.

~ Sarah

I eat small meals all day as opposed to three big meals. Also, I have fruit if I have dessert.
Good Luck!
~ Penny

Poker Chips instead of Potato Chips!
I have found a fun way to keep up with eating well and other healthy habits.   I found cheap colored poker chips in the dollar section of Target. I started with 2 Fruit chips, 1 Veggie, 2 Water, 2 Exercise (each chip equals 15 min. of exercise), 2 Dairy chips, Vitamins, and such. I also made some for my children. We each have a different color. When we have had that item, we put the chip in a jar and count them at the end of the day.

When the kids get to 200 points (about 2 weeks of doing 85% of the chips, they can see a movie, play games at

Chuck E. Cheese, etc.) The kids also have Chore chips, Homework chips and Hang up Clothes chips. I have also added 2 more Exercise chips (for a total of one hour per day) and am up to 6 water chips.
~ *Maureen*

My food secret: I realized at the age of 8 that I hated that "too full" feeling and have since only eaten to that "just satisfied" point.
~ *Sooze* (and her princess Alix)

I'm not thin now but here are things that I realize were different in my life when I was. Food was not a priority it was secondary to other things I had to do. I was not constantly sleep deprived when I was thin! If I was tired I got to rest. I didn't have to keep pushing because a family had needs that needed to be met whether I was tired or NOT!!
~ *Corinne*

I love to exercise and so does my husband. We belong to a health club and have for years. We also hike, bike, ski, play tennis, golf and swim. Our three kids are very active also. I don't buy processed foods except for bread. We don't eat out much, because it's not in our budget.
~ *Mary Fran*

My trick is simple: I decided that whatever the food industry says a serving should be, is plenty, and I get a serving or less out and put the rest away before I take a bite so I won't be tempted to have just a "little" more. Two added benefits are that I know exactly how much I ate, and I don't accidentally eat too much (except at buffets... there are no labels there!). My weight stays within a five pound range all the time this way, even though I rarely exercise.
~ *Tina*

I got fat after having four children and decided one day when I went to buy new underwear and had to buy the next size up again, that I didn't want to live this way. That was 20 years ago. (I had to think about how long ago it was.) It's a lifestyle.

~ Jesse

I'm a thin person. I LOVE food, how it smells, tastes and feels in my mouth. I try to eat things with flavors I really like and enjoy them.

~ Elisa

I Eat quality food, not quantity!

~ Kathleen

I mute all fast food commercials, rarely go to fast food places, and bypass the snack aisle at the grocery store. My inner child, SiAm, has accepted this lifestyle quite well after a number of years and only occasionally tries to dissuade me.

~ Dianne

I received your request today, and immediately thought of my LITTLE sister. She's 18 months younger than me, and we're polar opposites in size. She wore a girl's size 10 all through high school, and was back into those same clothes within 3 months of having her first baby. Here's her answer:

"I guess the first thing that popped into my head was 'Food is a necessary evil.' Seriously though, I eat when I'm hungry and stop when I'm not, and try to go for the healthiest food around unless I'm craving something specific."

I hope what my sister had to say helps. It's an interesting concept, to stop eating when you're not hungry anymore

(instead of when you're full, like I've always done). I know it's been said a million times, but I might actually try it now!
~ *Coral*

I have been thin most of my life...not a rail. I grew up with good food, before the fast food rush. I don't buy much trash to have in the house, but I have an occasional treat...ice cream, etc. I like small portions; that has begun to mean I eat out less because the plates are so huge and full. I lived in New Orleans for a longtime, where eating is entertainment. I had to get over that view. Buy healthy, don't keep lots in the house...few snacks in between meals. Thanks...

I'm a chef and I love food, however I knew when I went into the field I didn't want to end up like most of my colleagues, so I made it a habit NOT to eat while I'm cooking. Of course I taste as I create new dishes, but a taste doesn't have to be larger than a ¼ teaspoon.
~ *Karin*

Okay, kids, that's just a small selection of the hundreds of emails I got from thin people! I love the simplicity of some of their thoughts. Be careful with the "word" thin and think more about being healthy and adorable.

The most important thing is, as you play with my new ideas, you will gradually develop the mind of a person who is not preoccupied with food and therefore loving her life more.

Assignment for Chapter Ten:

Think adorable.

Start Body Shopping.

Go back and re-read the book chapter by chapter.

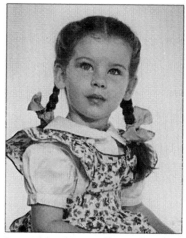

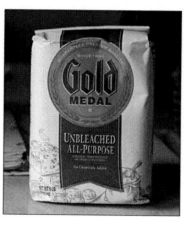

I use this picture of me when I was five, to remind me of Nelly my inner child.

My AHA moment came when I realized five pounds of flour was heavy.

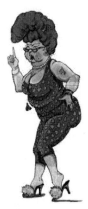

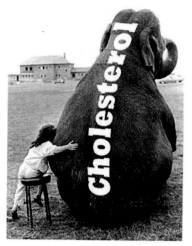

Katherine is my alter-ego. She reminds me to remember what it is I REALLY want. She's the part of me that came up with the line: "My mouth gets me into more trouble than any other hole in my body."

Cholesterol is our FRIEND!

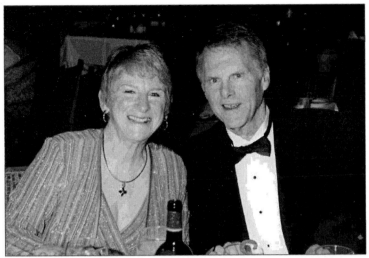

Terry and me on Jimmy Moore's low-carb cruise on "elegant" night. We are healthy and happy celebrating one year of being "low-carbers."

Remember, this is a vegetarian!

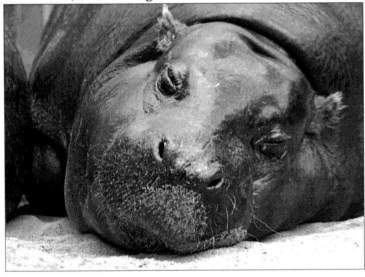

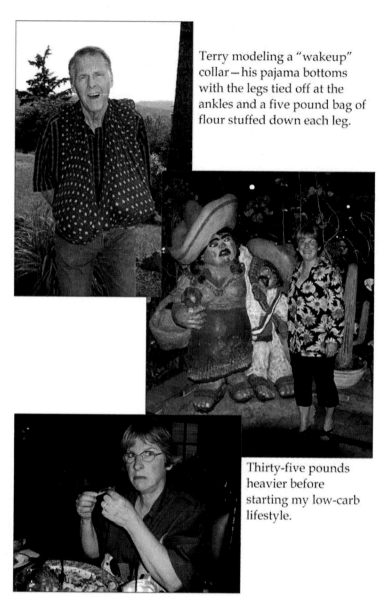

Terry modeling a "wakeup" collar—his pajama bottoms with the legs tied off at the ankles and a five pound bag of flour stuffed down each leg.

Thirty-five pounds heavier before starting my low-carb lifestyle.

Calories-in calories-out does not make for a happy girl!

Appendix

Weekly Progress Report
Self-discipline is remembering what you REALLY want.

GOAL

WEEK #		

YOUR RULES	INNER KIDDY'S REASONS	REWARD

Day/Date   What Happened Today?

GOAL RESULT _____

©2012 Pamela I Young

Grade for the week

Print copies of this report for free at the Make It Fun website,
www.makeitfunanditwillgetdone.com/mouthtrapdocs

Good Girl Report

Make it fun and it will get done!

Food	Carbs

Running Good Girl Total _____

Print copies of this report for free at the Make It Fun website,
www.makeitfunanditwillgetdone.com/mouthtrapdocs

Consumer Report

Make it fun and it will get done!

DATE _____   Carbs _____

Breakfast _____   _____

_____   _____

_____   _____

_____   _____

_____   _____

                                    TOTAL   _____

Lunch

_____   _____

_____   _____

_____   _____

_____   _____

_____   _____

                                    TOTAL   _____

Dinner

_____   _____

_____   _____

_____   _____

_____   _____

_____   _____

                                    TOTAL   _____

                          GRAND TOTAL   _____

Print copies of this report for free at the Make It Fun website,
www.makeitfunanditwillgetdone.com/mouthtrapdocs

Epilogue

December 6, 2010

While flying to Boston for Christmas, the first edition of this book was finished and was being polished by my wonderful editor Lorna Moon who had lost more than I had since she's been editing my manuscript.

The alarm went off at 4:00 am. The shuttle picked us up at 4:30 and we boarded the jet at 7:00. We were concerned that with the added security, check-in would take two hours. We zipped through in 10 minutes. We played cards and drank coffee until our flight was called.

Portland, Oregon to Boston on Alaska Airlines is a non-stop flight and we always try to up-grade to first class. We lucked out and were able to sit in row 3, seats A and B. Basking in the luxury of the big leather seats, I closed my eyes until we were at 30,000 feet. At 8:00 o'clock I was hungry since I'd been up since 4:00. I drank some water and waited for breakfast.

It had been over a year since we'd flown first class and instead of all the cutbacks I'd heard about, we were served a wonderful meal on small plates. I couldn't eat the whole breakfast. That said it all! I had changed not only on the outside, but the life behind my eyes had changed to match. It had taken love of my humanness, kindness and compassion for my inner child when I'd faltered to get where I was. I'd gained more than I'd lost. I'd lost the weight, but I'd gained the knowledge that my problem was absolutely a window to knowing and loving who I am.

After we landed and headed for baggage claim, I started noticing signs of Christmas in the airport terminal in

Boston. Over the speaker I heard Karen Carpenter singing *Have Yourself a Merry Little Christmas* in that golden voice that captured all of us years ago and continues to each Christmas season. I got tears in my eyes as I thought about Karen. She and her brother Richard were known as the *Carpenters* and were always part of every Christmas as their music is filled with joy and love for the season.

Beautiful Karen died in 1983 at the age of 33. She was anorexic. I think of her death when I hear that Christmas song for the first time each year. I still carry enough stored grief in her name to bring the tears, but this time I talked to her in my mind.

"Oh sweet Karen, I wish you could still be here sharing your gift with us. We miss you. You would still be here if you could only have known your eating problem was a window to love who you are."

The world lost Karen Carpenter to an eating disorder. Any disorder can be reversed with wellbeing. Wellbeing is widespread on this planet, but we tend to focus on what's gone wrong. We make news of it and turn it into various forms of official gossip. We don't need to do this. If the news upsets you, stop watching it. The news is just a soap opera and most of what we see; we can do nothing about. What we can do is practice living in wellbeing now right where we are.

My dear sweet listener and friend, love who you are. Be easy with yourself. Know that you are adored just as you are in this moment and in every moment. As you gradually change life-long habits, enjoy each phase of your transformation. You didn't get into your predicament in a week, month or even a year, so don't expect to get out of it in a shorter period of time. Take your time. You and your lovable inner child can do this if you stick together and refuse to allow anyone to cause you to doubt your ability to be in control of your magnificent mouth.

Enjoy!

Acknowledgements

I have to begin my acknowledgements by giving major credit to our tongues! They don't get much consideration unless we have a sore in our mouth or a chipped tooth and then we notice it because it keeps going to the trouble spot to check on it. The only other time it gets noticed is when one of those bud thingees gets upset and sticks up especially, when it's on the tip of our tongue. Tongues are the most exquisite creations. They work two very different occupations. One is blue collar and one is white. I talked about the assembly line work it does helping us to process food, but then it's almost like Clark Kent when he goes into a phone booth and comes out as Superman. If our tongue is Clark Kent on the assembly line, all we need to do is tell it we want to say something and it turns into this amazing organ that forms our speech with all the intricate sounds we learned when we were babies in order to use language. I am honored to know my tongue and I want to express my gratitude for all tongues across this beautiful planet of ours.

In the three years it has taken me write this book, lose 35 pounds and maintain it, Gary Taubes has been my inspiration. If it were not for his book *Why We Get Fat and What to do About it*, I would be struggling with the old calories-in, calories-out theory which is just plain wrong. Thank you Gary from the bottom of my heart. I know if I ever get to meet you, I'll gush like a teenage groupie.

Thank you to Marla Cilley who sent me *Why We Get Fat and What to do About it* as a gift.

I'd like to a give special thank you to Jimmy Moore for his selfless help for those who want to follow the low-carb lifestyle and Tom Naughton for bringing humor and information to us in Fat Head the documentary. I'm honored to have Dr. Ann Childers as my low carb physician who is on the cutting edge of the science of eating a high fat, restricted carbohydrate diet. She is an example of a beautiful, healthy woman who has been living this lifestyle for almost a decade.

Thank you to Lorna Moon, my editor for her inspiration and creativity. Because of her relationship with her inner child she is losing weight and looking great.

Thank you to Shannon Tracy my next door neighbor who graciously agreed to be on the cover of my book. (I had to swear to her the mouse trap had never been used.)

Thank you to Douglas Heidland my webmaster who is also an artist and designed the cover and did the layout for my book.

Thank you to Nelly my co-author who has filled my life with childlike joy and playfulness. I love you!

Thank you to all the wonderful small farmers who respect animals and the earth and supply us with healthy meats free of hormones and antibiotics and vegetables free of pesticides. Their work is a labor of love.

Last but not least, thank you to my husband Terry my soul mate, who has been there every step of the way in order to make this book a reality. And who loves me no matter what size I am.

Pam Young has been a reformed slob for more than 35 years. She teaches with humor and insight and her audiences take away creative strategies and practical steps to self-improvement in whatever area they choose.

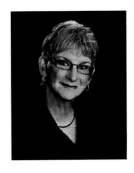

In 1977 Pam and her sister Peggy Jones decided they simply had to get organized and in the process found themselves with a business that has helped hundreds of thousands of disorganized women around the world and across at least two generations.

After writing six best-selling books together, being on thousands of radio and television shows, and speaking to audiences of thousands, Peggy retired in 2002. In addition to running their original business, Sidetracked Home Executives Inc., Pam decided to take her creativity and delightful sense of humor and launch the very popular website www.makeitfunanditwillgetdone.com to help a new generation of SHEs.

The Make it Fun website follows Pam's mission to be a positive force for good on the internet by striving to make this world a happier place through kind words, laughter, gentle direction and appreciation to women who seek to have their homes be peaceful, cozy, clean happy retreats from the world.

Based on innumerable SHE requests for Pam and Peggy's out of print best-selling book *The Sidetracked Sister's Happiness File*, Pam re-released it as an audio book in 2008. Listeners delighted in hearing Pam read the book and due to the overwhelming response the book was released as an eBook in 2009.

A challenge came to write a funny book about finances and Pam's initial reaction was, "Eegad, I'm in debt no way can I write that!" But after getting out of debt she wrote The GOOD Book: Get Out of Debt. Because of the success of the Happiness File audio book, Pam recorded the GOOD Book with all of her charm and wit. You'll find these books along with many great tools for being organized on her website.

Beyond being a best-selling author and home organizer, Pam's creativity is limitless. After finding an absolutely perfect artist in Diana Bonin, the two of them set to work and came up with a fun, funny and creative way to give cash gifts. If you have not seen Stick It Right on the Money Gift Kit you must go to the Make it Fun website and see Pam give a demonstration.

Of course, whatever Pam is doing you know there will be lots of smiles and laughter. How can there not be when Pam and Nelly's slogan is *Make it fun and it will get done*?